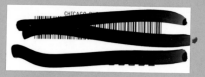

Practical Echocardiography and Doppler

Practical Echocardiography and Doppler

Mark J. Monaghan

Department of Cardiology
King's College Hospital
Denmark Hill, London

JOHN WILEY & SONS

Chichester · New York · Brisbane · Toronto · Singapore

Published 1990 by John Wiley & Sons Ltd.
Baffins Lane, Chichester
West Sussex PO19 1UD, England

Distributed in the United States of America,
Canada and Japan by Alan R. Liss Inc.,
41 East 11th Street, New York, NY 10003, USA.

Other Wiley Editorial Offices

John Wiley & Sons, Inc., 605 Third Avenue,
New York, NY 10158-0012, USA

Jacaranda Wiley Ltd, G.P.O. Box 859, Brisbane,
Queensland 4001, Australia

John Wiley & Sons (Canada) Ltd, 22 Worcester Road,
Rexdale, Ontario M9W 1L1, Canada

John Wiley & Sons (SEA) Pte Ltd, 37 Jalan Pemimpin #05-04,
Block B, Union Industrial Building, Singapore 2057

Library of Congress Cataloging-in-Publication Data:

Monaghan, Mark J.
    Practical echocardiography and doppler / Mark J. Monaghan.
        p.   cm.
    Includes bibliographies and index.
    ISBN 0 471 92069 X
    1. Echocardiography.   2. Heart—Diseases—Diagnosis
    I. Title.
    [DNLM: 1. Cardiovascular Diseases—diagnosis.
    2. Echocardiography—methods.   WG 141.5.E2 M734e]
RC683.5.U5M66   1989
616.1'207543—dc20
DNLM/DLC   89-14695
for Library of Congress   CIP

British Library Cataloguing in Publication Data:

Monaghan, Mark J.
    Practical echocardiography and doppler.
    1. Man. Heart. Diagnosis. Echocardiography
    I. Title
    616.1'207543

    ISBN 0 471 92069 X

Printed and bound in Great Britain by BAS Printers Ltd, Over Wallop, Hampshire

Contents

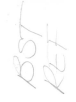

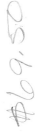

Foreword

Anyone who has attempted to perform an echocardiographic or Doppler examination knows that the beginning is most difficult. I know, for in the late 1960s I struggled with an M-Mode transducer for six months, trying to find my mitral valve. Only a few articles had been written on the subject at that time, no books existed. One night I was tired and I rolled onto my left side, and there was the valve!

When I was younger, I knew that echo techniques were likely to have importance for patient care. Indeed, nearly twenty years later, aside from routine chest X-ray and cineagiography, no technique for imaging the heart has had greater impact than echocardiography and Doppler. These ultrasound methods can now be used to establish a diagnosis and follow many cardiac disorders. In fact, their proper use may obviate the need for invasive procedures and serve as a principal means of directing the clinical decision-making process. Used in this way, a diagnosis may be quickly established with certainty, a patient's risk of physical harm reduced, and health care systems provided with a means of controlling cost.

Echocardiographic and Doppler systems are now widely available. Modestly priced relative to their benefit, such systems are now finding their way beyond large referral institutions and into primary care centers such as small hospitals, clinics and physician's offices. Many have learned that a diagnosis well made, or a possible diagnosis excluded with certainty, enhances our care of patients with cardiovascular disease.

This volume is aptly titled *Practical Echocardiography and Doppler*. Indeed, Mr Monaghan's approach is to be just that, *practical*. Only someone of his long experience, capability and internationally recognized stature could have produced such a volume. Mr. Monaghan developed an early desire to perfect the use of his modality. If only this volume existed during my early experience I would have saved six months of agonal self-experimentation.

Many books have been written about cardiac ultrasound techniques but most fail to deal with the practical issues: how to conduct a proper examination, how to judge quality, and what are the "tricks" used to optimize a diagnostic evaluation in certain disease states. Most books, in fact, begin with a ponderous chapter about how systems work and then jump immediately into complex diagnoses, failing to integrate technique with diagnosis. This book is different!

Mr Monaghan recognizes that echo and Doppler are methods requiring integration of the hand with the eye. He uses his considerable teaching skills and experience to build each chapter on the practical aspects of arriving at quality information. There are examples of various disease states. In addition, there are useful hints about how to obtain such examples. Some hints are tailored to specific disease states. All integrate use of the electronic equipment to produce the final result.

It is clear that this volume is the product of an individual who recognizes that good diagnostic data is the result of careful, but efficiently conducted examinations. The useful information contained in this volume will be helpful to those at any level of experience, but those just beginning will find it the most useful.

Mr Monaghan is recognized internationally as a learned teacher of these methods. I am privileged by my long association with him, both professionally and personally. As anyone who thoughtfully interacts with the contents of this book will see, I continue to learn from him. Moreover, it is the patients we encounter who ultimately benefit.

Joseph Kisslo, MD
Professor of Medicine
Duke University Medical Center
Durham, North Carolina, USA

Preface

Some fifteen years ago, Dr Peter Richardson, who is a cardiologist in our department, invited me to look into the enclosed hood of a new diagnostic instrument called an echocardiograph. In front of my eyes passed some strange hieroglyphics that looked as though they had been produced by some ancient cave dweller! He reliably informed me that these waveforms sweeping across the front of the oscilloscope were produced by the small transducer on the patient's chest and were derived from sound pulses bouncing off the mitral valve. From that moment on I was hooked. It seemed to me that a bedside technique that was completely noninvasive and yet able to provide such dynamic information about intracardiac structures had to have a very important future in cardiology. I have a lot to thank Peter for, because since that first introduction to echocardiography I have found the technique completely absorbing and fascinating. It has clearly expanded beyond our wildest dreams, and just as one thinks a plateau has been reached in the development of the technique, a new technical innovation or clinical application appears around the corner. I am confident that echocardiography and Doppler will continue to be the most important tools in noninvasive diagnostic cardiology for many years to come. I hope that some of my obsessional enthusiasm for these techniques will rub off on the readers of this book.

The book has certainly had a long gestation. It was many years ago that I realized that very few of the texts on echo dealt with the practical aspects of the technique and showed how, in a straightforward manner, to perform the examination and arrive at the correct diagnosis. I naively put pen to paper thinking that it would be relatively easy to describe those same methods that I taught during lectures and demonstrated during my echo sessions. It was certainly more protracted and difficult than I ever imagined and the manuscript has been through many revisions. I am indebted to all those people who by their persistent badgering persuaded me to complete this task. I also owe thanks to those I have taught over the years; through trial and error I have learned from them the right and wrong ways to teach these very practical techniques. Do not imagine for one moment that by reading this book you will be able to perform echocardiography and Doppler; it will also take many long hours learning how to put into practice the theory contained in these pages. But I promise you will enjoy learning!

This book is dedicated to four people—my wife Fran and sons James, Thomas and Guy. They have spent many evenings and weekends alone whilst I formed a close relationship with a word processor! I owe them thanks for their patience and encouragement and I hope that both they and you feel that the result has been worthwhile.

Mark J. Monaghan

Abbreviations

A.AO	=	ascending aorta
AML	=	anterior mitral valve leaflet
AO	=	aorta
ARCH	=	aortic arch
AV	=	aortic valve
CL	=	closure line
D.AO	=	descending aorta
EFF	=	effusion
ET	=	ejection time (may be derived from simultaneous carotid pulse recording)
IAS	=	interatrial septum
IVS	=	interventricular septum
JVP	=	jugular venous pressure
LA	=	left atrium
LC	=	left coronary aortic valve cusp/leaflet
LMCA	=	left main coronary artery
LV	=	left ventricle
LVed	=	left ventricular end-diastolic dimension
LVes	=	left ventricular end-systolic dimension
LVOT	=	left ventricular outflow tract
LVPW	=	left ventricular posterior wall
MPA	=	main pulmonary artery
MV	=	mitral valve
NC	=	noncoronary aortic valve cusp/leaflet
PA	=	pulmonary artery
PASP	=	pulmonary artery systolic pressure
PM	=	papillary muscle
PML	=	posterior mitral valve leaflet
PV	=	pulmonary valve
RA	=	right atrium
RASP	=	right atrial systolic pressure
RC	=	right coronary aortic valve cusp/leaflet
RV	=	right ventricle
RVOT	=	right ventricular outflow tract
RVSP	=	right ventricular systolic pressure
TGC	=	time-gain compensation
TV	=	tricuspid valve
VCF	=	mean circumferential fiber shortening velocity
Veg	=	vegetation
VSD	=	ventricular septal defect

CHAPTER 1

Basic physics and technology of echocardiography

This chapter will concentrate only on those essential aspects of physics and technology that are necessary to have an understanding of the principles of echocardiography, its limitations and potential.

Important design features of modern echo machines and the operation of instrument controls will also be discussed and interrelated with physical principles where relevant.

Relevant aspects of Doppler instrumentation are discussed in Chapter 11.

The transducer – how ultrasound is generated and detected

Bats use ultrasound to visualize their environment in a similar manner to the way echocardiography images the heart. Ultrasound is, of course, very high frequency sound and is above the limit of human hearing which is approximately 20 kHz. In echocardiography, frequencies of between 1.5 MHz and 7.5 MHz are currently used.

There is a direct relationship between the velocity of the sound waves, their frequency and their wavelength. In soft tissues (e.g. the heart) the velocity of sound is 1540 m/s. This means that at 7.5 MHz the wavelength is 0.2 mm whereas at 1.5 MHz the wavelength is approximately 1.0 mm. The wavelength of the sound used determines the potential of the technique to resolve small structures and therefore, to a certain extent, the resolution.

Unfortunately, higher frequency sound waves are more easily absorbed and diffracted by tissue interfaces. So, while high frequencies may give better resolution, they have poor penetration and will not provide satisfactory images of deep structures. Therefore high frequencies (5 MHz and above) tend to be used more for pediatric imaging where great penetration is not required. If a choice of transducers is available, then the highest frequency that provides adequate penetration should be used. If a Doppler examination is being performed, then lower frequencies are more suitable as described in Chapter 11.

Ultrasound is generated by a physical principle known as the piezoelectric effect. If an electrical voltage is applied across opposite faces of a piezoelectric material then the material will physically expand or contract depending upon the polarity of the applied voltage, as shown in Figure 1.1.

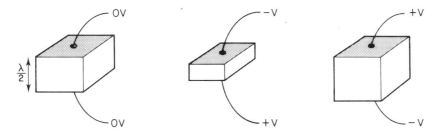

Figure 1.1 Piezoelectric crystal with electrodes bonded onto alternate surfaces and their appropriate electrical connections. The crystal is manufactured to be one half wavelength thickness of the desired ultrasound frequency. When an electrical charge is placed across the crystal surfaces (through the electrodes) the crystal shape is deformed and it will oscillate at a predetermined frequency. Alternatively, when the crystal is itself deformed by sound waves it will produce a voltage on the electrodes which can be detected.

If the voltage is applied as a short pulse, the crystal will immediately deform and then oscillate in size for a period, ringing rather like a "dinner-gong" struck with a hammer. The frequency of the oscillation is mainly determined by the thickness of the piezoelectric material. A transducer of a particular frequency is made by cutting the piezoelectric material to a half wavelength thickness of the desired oscillation frequency. Thus to manufacture an ultrasound transducer that would produce 5 MHz centre frequency ultrasound, the crystal would have to be cut 0.15 mm thick.

As the piezoelectric material oscillates (expanding and contracting) it produces high and low pressure waves, i.e. sound waves. The actual piezoelectric materials used in ultrasound imaging are crystals of barium titanate or lead zirconate titanate. Electrodes are bonded onto opposing surfaces of the crystal to apply and detect the electrical signals.

If sound waves of the appropriate frequency strike a piezoelectric crystal, it will tend to mechanically oscillate and resonate at that frequency. As it does so, it will itself generate an electrical voltage across its surfaces that can be detected by the electrodes. This means we can use the same crystal both to generate ultrasound waves of a desired frequency and also to detect them. The crystal will detect sound of any frequency but is much more sensitive to sound of the same frequency that it produces.

Design and construction of an ultrasound transducer is a very expensive and exacting process. The ultrasound has to be generated and propagated into the tissues as efficiently as possible, with minimum energy losses and with the width of the ultrasound beam kept as narrow as possible (to maximize resolution). The same transducer must be able to receive and detect the ultrasound in an efficient and sensitive manner with a minimum of artefacts.

As ultrasound travels through the tissues, some of it is reflected back towards the transducer as an echo every time the sound crosses an interface. In the heart these reflecting interfaces are typically the junctions between blood and the heart valves or myocardial tissue. At every interface some sound is reflected back and the remainder travels further into the tissue until the next interface. The strength of the returning echo is dependent upon the difference in acoustic impedance (density) of the two materials at the interface and also the angle at which the sound strikes the interface. Thus strong echoes are generated by dense interfaces (e.g. calcified valves) that are oriented perpendicular to the sound beam.

Since the same transducer crystal is used both to transmit and receive the ultrasound, the sound is generated in pulses. A short pulse of ultrasound is transmitted (containing a few wavelengths) and the transducer then detects the returning echoes from the various interfaces. Since the speed of the sound pulse is virtually constant within soft tissue, the instrument can display the distance between the transducer and the interfaces by timing how long it takes the echoes

to return after the pulse is transmitted. The intensity of the returning echo is also displayed in terms of a gray scale.

Since the time taken to generate an echo pulse and reflect it back from a distance of say 20 cm is so short, it is possible to sample all interface distances within that range approximately 1000 times/second. Therefore, not only can distances be appreciated but also the motion of structures.

The transmit or output control

If the piezoelectric crystal is allowed to continue ringing like the "dinner-gong" then a very long sound pulse will be produced. This will contain a lot of energy and therefore generate strong bright echoes. However, if the pulse is longer than the distance between two separate interfaces, then the echoes from the interfaces will merge together and be detected as one. Thus long pulses will reduce the resolution of imaging and limit our ability to visualize separately structures that are positioned close together.

The length of the ultrasound pulse is usually controlled by a transmit or output control which regulates how long the crystal rings to produce each pulse. Since this reflects how much energy is contained in the pulse, this control may be calibrated in terms of decibels (dB). The control is adjusted to provide images that are of adequate brightness throughout the entire image plane without compromising resolution. Structures such as the pericardium and calcified or prosthetic valves should have a maximum (white) gray level, the blood-filled cavities should be almost echo free (black), and the myocardium should, under normal circumstances, have a mid gray level. As the transmit control is increased the myocardium becomes brighter, a speckled artefact may appear in the cavities, and individual echoes appear larger as the resolution decreases.

The compress or reject control

All ultrasound images contain some noise signals. These are usually of a low level and may be ultrasound artefacts or electrical noise generated in the image processing circuits. Since the presence of this noise is distracting and undesirable in an image, it can be removed (if it is of low intensity) by the use of the compress or reject control.

This control essentially cuts out all signals below a certain level. It is optimally adjusted so that as much low level noise is removed from the image without rejecting excessive real image data. This can be done by ensuring that the blood-filled cavities do not contain too many low level echoes and that thin, weak reflecting structures such as normal

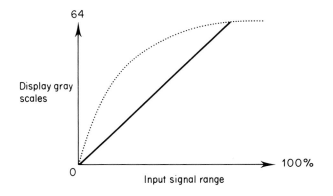

Figure 1.2 Graphical representation of how the input signal range (0–100%) can be mapped onto display gray scales in different ways. The continuous line demonstrates a linear transfer function, whereas the dotted line shows a processing curve in which most of the gray scales are allocated to lower intensity signals. Mid- to high-range signals are all compressed into the top few gray scales. If a reject control is used, gray levels below the reject level are all displayed as black, whereas a compress control utilizes (at all times) the entire gray level range.

aortic valve leaflets are not cut out of the image. In many patients, a compromise between the settings of the transmit and the compress controls has to be achieved to obtain the best possible image, therefore some experience in operating the equipment is required.

There is a subtle but important difference between the way that a compress and a reject control actually work. With equipment using reject, all gray levels below the reject level are not displayed in the image and will be black. Therefore, the range of gray levels displayed will be from above the reject level through to white. The compress control redistributes the entire gray level range in the image (from black to white) to those echo signals which are above the compress level. So while both types of controls allow the operator to remove signals below a certain level, compress makes most efficient use of the available gray levels by ensuring that the entire gray scale is always used (see Figure 1.2).

Image processing

After low level noisy signals have been removed using reject or compress, the remaining data has to be assigned into gray levels to make up the image. The range of signal intensities at this stage is typically 100 000 : 1. Most video display screens can only cope with a maximum of 64 separate shades of gray level. Therefore there has to be considerable compression of the original data to fit into a 64 : 1 display

range. This is in part one of the functions of the compress control.

The way in which this translation into levels occurs can be controlled using a variety of image processing or transfer functions which are available on most instruments. The simplest way to perform this translation is with a linear relationship between the signal intensity and the resultant gray level. However, there are occasions when it is more useful to use a curved or an S shape transfer function as shown in Figure 1.2. For example, if a certain range of input signal levels is required to occupy more of the gray levels or if high level signals are to be reduced in the image, then nonlinear transfer would be used. Examples of this are shown in Figure 1.2. In basic terms, altering the image processing can appear to make the image softer, or increase the contrast, or boost a specific range of echoes.

Image processing of this type can occur at different stages and may also be used to manipulate the appearance of images played back from a video recorder into the machine. These controls are often called pre- and post-processing. Reference should be made to the manufacturer's guide for exact nomenclature and suggested settings.

Gain controls

The echo signals received by the instrument are extremely weak and must be amplified before translation into gray levels. In addition, echoes received from distant structures are many times weaker than those returning from the near field. This is because at every interface the ultrasound pulse loses energy due to partial reflection (the returning echoes) and also absorption losses. Therefore it is necessary to amplify those echoes received from the far field to a greater extent.

In most ultrasound systems there is a control system that allows for a variation in gain over the depth of the image. This is usually known as time-gain compensation (TGC) or depth-gain control. One of the most straightforward arrangements for TGC is a series of separate (often slider) gain controls. Each control adjusts the amplification of signals returning from a particular depth range and facilitates quite easy and detailed control of the image intensity over the entire depth of field. With these controls, the gain is usually adjusted to a low setting in the near field of the image, is increased in the mid field and may be reduced again at the depth of the pericardium since this is a strong echo reflector.

An alternative arrangement is with one control that adjusts signal gain over the entire image. This is set so that structures in the far field have satisfactory image intensity. A separate control allows further adjustment to near field signals. This control is usually set to a lower level. The transition from near field gain control to overall image gain is achieved with an adjustable ramp which can be altered in terms of both depth position and rate of gain increase.

In practical terms both these methods of variable gain adjustment achieve similar results and their precise method of operation will differ between manufacturers.

Depth control

The use of this control is virtually self-explanatory. The scan depth can usually be varied, in fixed stages, over a range from approximately 4 cm to a maximum of 25 cm. The required depth setting is chosen so that the cardiac structures fill the entire image area and unwanted, deeper structures do not occupy the image.

It does take a finite time for an ultrasound pulse to travel to the desired maximum depth and return to the transducer: this is the time required to construct one scan line of data (see next section). There is a trade-off between the scan depth, the scan rate and the scan line density, scan line density being the relationship between the number of individual scan lines of data in an image and the scan angle (usually 90°). To optimize all the above factors it is important that the minimum practical depth setting is used every time. On some instruments, factors such as the scan (frame) rate are displayed and the effect of changing the depth setting can be seen.

With some transducer systems it is possible to adjust the focus of the ultrasound beam electronically. When the instrument depth setting is changed, the beam focus is altered to provide optimum resolution at about halfway down the image. It is therefore essential to ensure that the depth control is adjusted correctly.

Chart recorder speed

This is usually adjustable from speeds of 10 mm/s up to 100 mm/s. The actual speed used will often be a matter of personal preference or economics (since recording paper is very expensive). However, 50 mm/s is the most commonly used speed for M-Mode recordings. When it is required to study the timing of intracardiac events, a recording speed of 100 mm/s is more satisfactory. Calibration markers at 1 cm depth are recorded onto the paper at 1 s intervals and facilitate an easy method of confirming the recording speed. In order to optimize the quality of an individual image, all of the above instrument settings will require adjustment. The precise control settings required will depend upon the exact image plane being used and also the anatomy of the

patient. It is important to practice with these controls so their adjustment becomes as automatic as manipulating the transducer between the various image planes!

How the 2D image is created

For cardiac imaging we require a transducer system that will created a fan of ultrasound and therefore produce a wedge- or sector-shaped image. This is because the heart is a relatively large structure when compared with the size of the imaging window. The size of the window is limited by the ribs and lungs, both of which absorb and diffract the ultrasound signals. It is rather like looking through a keyhole into the room beyond.

There are usually about 120 scan lines (in a 90° sector image) creating the fan of ultrasound. Each line is created by sending a pulse down the line direction and then collecting all the reflected echoes from that line. Since sound travels relatively fast, each line can be built up quickly and a whole sector frame of 120 lines is created in about 1/30th of a second.

As previously mentioned, there is an obvious trade-off between the time taken to create an entire sector frame, the number of lines in the frame and the depth of scanning. All these factors are limited by the speed of sound in soft tissue, which is fixed at 1540 m/s. It is desirable to have as many lines of data in an image as possible since this improves resolution and therefore the appreciation of detailed and small structures. The time taken to create one sector frame should be as short as possible so that each image depicts the position of all structures at one moment in time. This is important because intracardiac structures such as valves move fast. In addition, if the time taken to create an individual image is short then the frame rate of the moving (real-time) images is high. This is necessary to avoid unpleasant and distracting image flicker. The human eye can detect this flicker if the frame rate drops much below 30 Hz.

There are a variety of methods currently used for steering the ultrasound pulses down individual scan lines to create the sector image. These methods can be divided into mechanical and electronic techniques, the former being both simpler and cheaper.

The most common two types of mechanically operated transducers are shown in Figures 1.3 and 1.4. In Figure 1.3 a rotating transducer is illustrated. This consists of three or four crystal piezoelectric elements mounted on a wheel which rotates in an oil bath. As an individual element rotates over the image area it fires pulses (one for each scan line) and detects the returning echoes from each line. As one element reaches the end of the sector, the next one is positioned to create a new sector with another series of

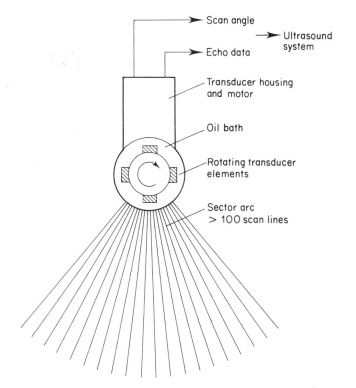

Figure 1.3 Diagram of a mechanical rotating sector transducer system. A rotating wheel within an oil bath has three or four piezoelectric elements attached to it. Each element is activated to produce ultrasound scan lines as it sweeps over the predetermined sector arc.

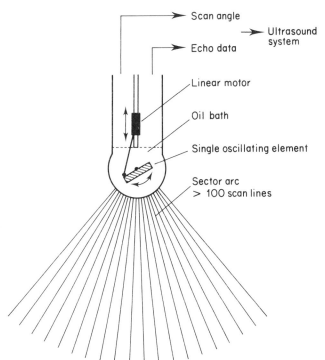

Figure 1.4 Diagram of a mechanical oscillatory transducer system. A single oscillating element positioned in an oil bath sweeps backwards and forwards over the sector arc.

scan lines. The echo signals from each line are fed back to the instrument together with precise information about the position of the element, i.e. which scan line the signals are coming from. This type of mechanical transducer tends to be relatively large because of the space required to accommodate the rotating wheel and piezoelectric elements.

The oscillatory type of mechanical transducer is shown in Figure 1.4. This transducer has a single piezoelectric element which is rapidly swept forwards and backwards through the sector arc by mechanical linkage to a linear motor. Throughout each sweep a series of scan lines are created and both the scan line data and position of the element are continuously fed back to the ultrasound system. This type of transducer tends to be relatively light, small and able to fit into small intercostal spaces.

Electronic beam steering can be achieved using phased array technology. This technique is very complicated and phased array transducers are expensive. However, this technique does have some advantages which are explained later. As illustrated in Figure 1.5a, the crystal element in this type of transducer is in fact divided up into a number of individual small elements. There are usually between 64 and 128 of these elements, with each one having separate electronic connections. When each of these elements is fired it creates a little wavefront of sound, rather like the ripples spreading out from a pebble dropped in a pond. The wavefronts from all the individual elements merge together at a distance of about 1 cm from the transducer to form a compound wave which travels away from the transducer.

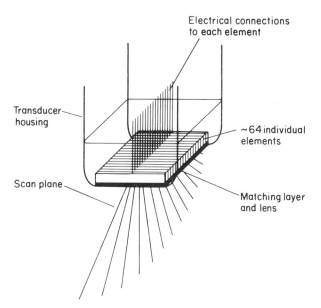

Figure 1.5a Diagram of a phased array transducer system, showing the transducer housing with the piezoelectric crystal positioned beneath the matching layer and lens on the transducer surface. The crystal is cut into 64 or 128 individual elements. Each element has separate electrical connections.

If all the elements are fired at exactly the same time, the compound wave travels in a direction exactly perpendicular to the transducer face, as shown in Figure 1.5b. If the elements are fired slightly out of sequence or phase with each other, the wave fronts merge to form a compound wave which is steered in a direction dependent on the firing sequence. By controlling very precisely the firing sequence of the elements, the compound wave (ultrasound pulse) can be steered in any direction, as illustrated in Figures 1.5c and 1.5d. The pulses are in fact fired in sequence down each of the scan lines that make up the image plane.

One advantage of this technique is that the beam is steered without using any moving parts; in theory at least this may make phased array transducers more reliable than

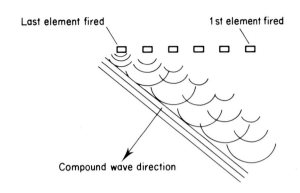

Figure 1.5d   The firing sequence is now arranged so that the compound wave is steered down another scan line in another direction.

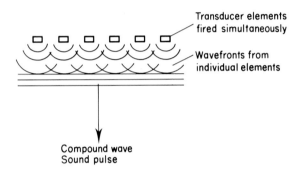

Figure 1.5b   Diagrammatic representation of multiple wavefronts emerging from six of the transducer elements which have been fired simultaneously. A short distance from the transducer, the individual wavefronts from each element merge together to produce a compound wave which travels directly away, perpendicular to the transducer face.

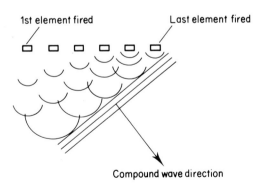

Figure 1.5c   Here the six elements have been fired out of phase with each other. When the individual wavefronts merge to form a compound wave it is not oriented parallel to the transducer face and therefore travels away at an angle. That angle can be altered by varying the phase lag between the firing of all the individual elements. Therefore, the ultrasound wave can be electronically steered down multiple separate scan lines by controlling the firing sequence of all the elements.

their mechanical counterparts, although the latter are easier to repair. The phased array technology is also used to focus the beam so that it is at its narrowest at any desired depth. Variable focusing is not possible on most mechanical transducer systems. In addition to focusing the transmitted beam, it is also possible to focus the receive part of the transducer system so that any one instant in time the transducer is selectively receiving only those echoes coming from a specified beam direction and depth. This is known as dynamic receive focusing and helps to reduce the effects of spurious ultrasound echoes which would cause artefacts on the image.

The resolution of phased array systems in the near field (at shallow depths) tends to be inferior to that of mechanical systems. This is because of "side lobes" which are small off-axis ultrasound beams produced by interaction between the individual elements. These side lobes produce artefacts that limit the imaging resolution, particularly at shallow depths. The electronic focusing techniques are very successful in reducing, although not completely eliminating, the effects of side lobes.

Annular array transducers are in effect a combination of both mechanical and phased array technologies. An example is seen in Figure 1.6. These transducers are constructed in a similar way to oscillatory transducers with a mechanically steered piezoelectric element. However, the circular element is divided into a number of individual, concentrically arranged ring elements that can be fired in sequence like a phased array transducer. This means that the transducer can be focused both on transmit and receive to ensure a very narrow beam and therefore high resolution. The beam itself is steered mechanically. The annular array technology theoretically combines some advantages of both mechanical and phased array systems.

The echo signals received by any of the transducer systems are converted into electrical impulses as previously described. These electrical impulses are fed back into the ultrasound system and used to construct the 2D image. The

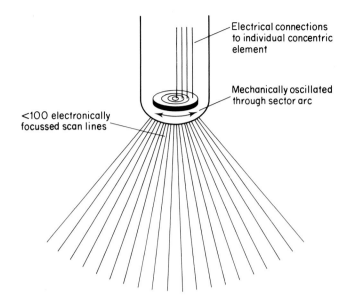

Figure 1.6 Diagram of an annular array transducer system. A single crystal is mechanically oscillated through the sector arc as in the oscillatory transducer system. However, the crystal is cut into individual concentric circles forming separate elements. These elements can be fired as in the phased array transducer. This is used to focus the sound beam so that it may be kept very narrow and reduces the possibility of beam width artefacts.

electrical impulses are in a continuously varying (analog) format and are converted into digital values to allow more convenient computer processing. Each electrical impulse (echo signal) is normally assigned to one of 64 (or 128) individual levels depending upon its intensity and the processing curve selected.

The radial scan lines now contain a number of digital gray level data points. To allow the images to be displayed on standard video monitors and recorded onto video tape the image has to be converted into a standard TV format. This format consists of horizontal lines rather than the original radial scan lines that made up the image. The transfer to TV format is performed by a digital scan converter. The scan converter is essentially a memory matrix which contains many individual image pixels (typically 600 × 400 pixels). These pixels are like tiny image building blocks – each of the pixels can be assigned a gray level and together they form the image in the scan converter. The pixels are also used to display alphanumeric data on the image such as the date, patient identification and tape numbers. The data in the pixels can be read out of the scan converter as a number of individual horizontal lines to make up the TV format. In addition, the image can be frozen in the scan converter, making it easy to calculate distances and areas etc.

The quality of the displayed image is very dependent on the scan converter. If there are too few pixels in the scan converter then the relative size of each pixel will be large and the image will have a rather blocky, jagged appearance

with the outline of each pixel quite obvious. Scan converters with a large number of very small pixels will produce smooth images that are detailed and pleasant to the eye; needless to say, the larger digital memory and also the increased image processing speed required increases the cost of these scan converters.

The exact way in which the scan converter assigns a particular level to a pixel also has a significant effect upon the image quality. As illustrated in Figure 1.7, a significant number of image pixels will not be placed in the same relative position as data points on the scan lines. There are also many more image pixels than data points in a typical scan converter. So a significant amount of interpolation must occur to give each pixel a gray level for every frame. In a simple scan converter this may be achieved by simply allocating that level which is found in the nearest data point on the scan lines. Sophisticated scan converters use a variety of algorithms (usually patented) to take into account the gray level values in all surrounding data points and their distances from the pixel. The more complicated algorithms produce images which are likely to be more realistic. However, since the levels in every pixel must be updated about 30 times a second, exceedingly fast and therefore relatively

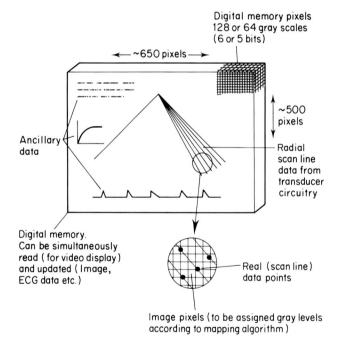

Figure 1.7 The digital scan converter, which converts radial scan line data from the transducer system into a digital memory matrix which can be frozen and also used to create the horizontal TV/video format. The scan converter is essentially a digital memory consisting of multiple elements each of which can be assigned a gray level. The scan converter will fill in gaps between the radial scan line data points to produce an attractive image and will also allow superimposition of ancillary data such as patient identification, processing curves, dates and ECG recordings.

expensive processors must be used. As we have seen in other aspects of ultrasound instrumentation, high image quality is more expensive to produce. However, this does not always explain the differences in costs of competing ultrasound equipment.

How the M-Mode record is created

The M-Mode or time motion recording is simply a graph of echo signal depths (down any single scan line) against time. The original M-Mode studies were performed using a single crystal transducer that was pointed in the desired direction. Modern equipment uses 2D transducers, the precise direction of the M-Mode beam being selected using a movable cursor that can be positioned over the image as shown in Figure 1.8. This is certainly more convenient and allows complete verification of the geometrical orientation of the M-Mode beam path to the cardiac anatomy.

When M-Mode is selected in any form of mechanical transducer system, the transducer element is precisely positioned and held stationary so that information is derived just from the selected M-Mode beam direction. This means that it is not possible to simultaneously acquire and display an M-Mode and a real-time (moving) 2D echo. Phased array transducer systems use no moving parts and therefore,

as previously described, it is possible for the transducer system to sample any of the scan lines, in any sequence, very rapidly. Therefore when M-Mode is selected the ultrasound system is able to time share between creating a real-time 2D image and a simultaneous M-Mode. For example, the M-Mode line is sampled, then the first line of the 2D image, then the M-Mode line again, then the second line of the 2D image and so on. Since the phased array ultrasound system is spending part of its time creating 2D images, the sampling frequency of the M-Mode line is less than with mechanical transducer systems. This appears to be more a theoretical than a practical disadvantage and in the author's opinion does not adversely affect the quality of the M-Mode recordings.

The ability to simultaneously display real-time M-Mode and 2D echoes does have some advantages, particularly in the initial stages of learning echocardiography and also when trying to achieve an M-Mode recording of a small structure such as the pulmonary valve. However, it is by no means an essential requirement.

The time sharing principle can be extended in some systems to allow two different M-Modes and simultaneous real-time 2D echoes to be collected. The sampling frequency of the M-Modes and the 2D will be clearly reduced in this mode and the technique does not appear to have a routine clinical application.

In order to achieve a pleasing and satisfactory M-Mode recording, the ultrasound data is processed in a slightly

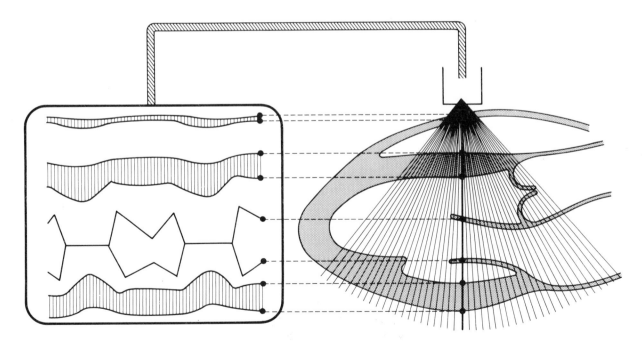

Figure 1.8   Creation of the M-Mode recording. A cursor can be moved over the 2D image to select the precise position of the M-Mode beam direction. Echo data from the selected line is then displayed on the screen as a graph of depth against time. Superimposed on top of this recording will be a calibration scale of depth (in centimeters) and time (in seconds). The M-Mode technique allows detailed evaluation of particular structures and is convenient for facilitating measurements.

different way to that normally used for 2D images. For example, most users prefer 2D images to have a black background with white tissue echoes, whereas M-Modes have traditionally had white backgrounds and black tissue echoes. From a diagnostic point of view it makes little difference; however, since 2D images are usually viewed on a video monitor and M-Modes as a paper recording, this arrangement is probably easier on the eye.

Although 2D images are digitally processed, this can be undesirable in M-Mode recordings since it leads to a blocky appearance. Therefore, most ultrasound systems provide an analog M-Mode. Edge enhancement processing is also often performed to give a slightly crisper appearance with clearly defined echo edges. Fewer gray scales tend to be used in M-Mode and this increases the contrast of the recordings. Most of these features and differences in M-Mode processing are incorporated because of user preference rather than any major diagnostic advantage.

CHAPTER 2

Scanning techniques

As discussed in Chapter 1, M-Mode recordings are obtained using a 2D image as a guide and reference to the selection of the beam direction. Therefore the techniques of 2D scanning are discussed first in this chapter.

Patient preparation

A large proportion of the general public are aware that ultrasound imaging techniques are both painless and completely safe. However, some patients, especially young children, will be apprehensive about the investigation that they are to undergo. It should go without saying that a brief explanation will pay dividends in terms of patient relaxation and cooperation.

All echocardiographic equipment will have facilities for recording physiological parameters such as an ECG simultaneously with the echo images. An ECG is certainly useful, although not essential. Limb electrode systems are more economical to use than disposable chest electrodes; however, the latter are more convenient.

Most patients will be easier to scan (using the left parasternal and apical imaging windows) if they are positioned in a left lateral decubitus position. This procedure tends to rotate the heart out from under the sternum. If the patient's left arm is raised with the hand behind the head the size of the parasternal window is also increased.

For subcostal imaging the patient should be semi-supine, preferably with the legs bent so that the abdomen is relaxed. To obtain satisfactory suprasternal images it is usually necessary to lay the patient as flat as possible on their back and place a pillow under the shoulders so that the head and neck are stretched back. This procedure increases transducer access to the suprasternal area. However, it can be quite uncomfortable and cooperation may be difficult to achieve in children and patients who are breathless when

lying flat. Therefore it is usually prudent to perform suprasternal imaging, if it is required, towards the end of the examination.

Calcified ribs in adults and older children are relatively impenetrable by ultrasound and may diffract it, causing shadows and artefacts on the images. This problem is largely circumvented by ensuring that the transducer is not positioned directly over ribs.

Most echocardiographers are familiar with the fact that lungs absorb ultrasound. If the lungs cover most of the heart, imaging can be extremely difficult. This tends to occur particularly in patients with chronic obstructive airways disease or emphysema and in heavy smokers. In these situations it is often helpful to get the patient to hold their breath in expiration for a few seconds while images are recorded. When performing subcostal imaging, held inspiration is preferable since this tends to push the heart inferiorly.

Transducer manipulation requires a certain amount of dexterity and hand-to-eye coordination. Therefore most echocardiographers find it easier to hold the transducer in almost the same way and using the same hand as a pen would normally be held. For the majority of people this will obviously be in the right hand. The left hand is then used to operate the instrument controls. There will be occasions, however, when space is limited and left-handed scanning is necessary. If possible, the arm being used for scanning should be supported and will often rest across the patient. This is very important since it reduces arm and back fatigue. It also limits the possibility of the transducer slipping unnoticed away from the imaging window, and reduces the pressure of the transducer on the chest.

Ultrasound gel has an important role to play in maintaining the quality of echo images. To a certain extent the gel acts as a lubricant to allow easy transducer movement over the chest wall. However, its main role is as a couplant and interface between the transducer face and the skin. It excludes air from this junction and has an acoustic impedance which is specifically designed to increase the efficiency of ultrasound transfer between the transducer and the chest. It is important to use sufficient thickness of gel so that, if the transducer is angled, gel still forms the "bridge" between the entire transducer face and the skin. For this reason, echocardiographic ultrasound gel has a higher viscosity (at room temperature) than the gels and oils used in other types of ultrasound scanning where the transducer face can more easily maintain contact with the skin.

Standard 2D image planes

Since 2D images are tomographic slices through the heart, these slices can be (and frequently are) made in an infinite number of different planes! In reality, the number of imaging planes normally used is limited by the access windows available. These are usually parasternal, apical, subcostal and suprasternal, as shown in Figure 2.1. There is also the obvious need to use standardized and internationally recognized 2D views and planes. The American Society of Echocardiography has defined a series of standardized

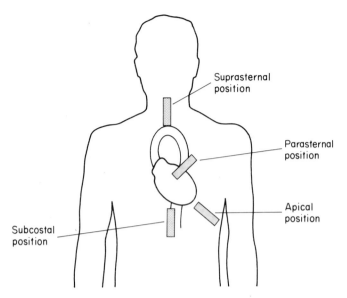

Figure 2.1 Transducer positions to obtain parasternal, apical, subcostal and suprasternal echo images.

imaging views which have achieved almost universal acceptance. These views and planes are illustrated in Figures 2.2 and 2.3.

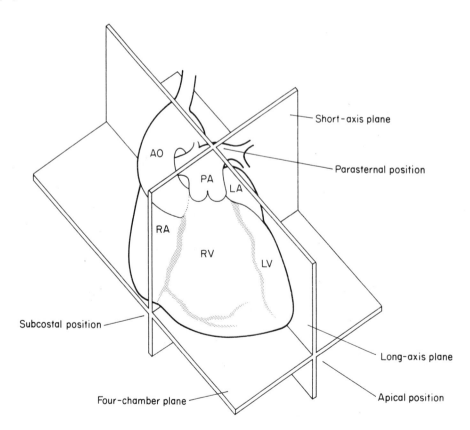

Figure 2.2 Diagram illustrating the relationship of the long axis, short axis and four chamber planes to the heart. Respective parasternal, apical and subcostal transducer positions are shown. By permission of the American Society of Echocardiography. Modified from the Report of the ASE Committee on Nomenclature and Standards in Two-Dimensional Echocardiography, August 1980.

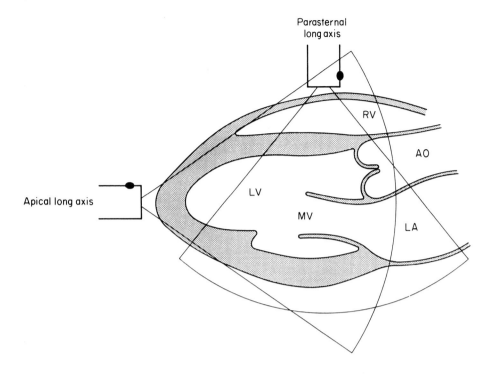

Figure 2.3a Long axis imaging plane which can be obtained from both parasternal and apical transducer positions.

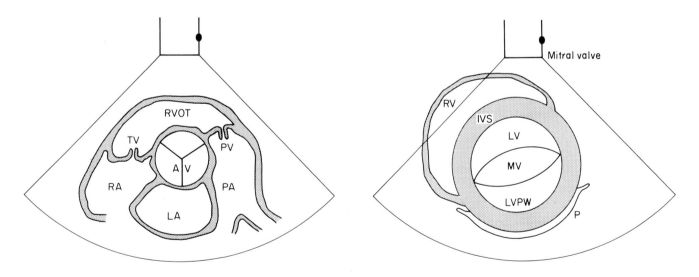

Figure 2.3b Parasternal short axis imaging plane at aortic valve level.

Figure 2.3c Parasternal short axis plane at mitral valve level.

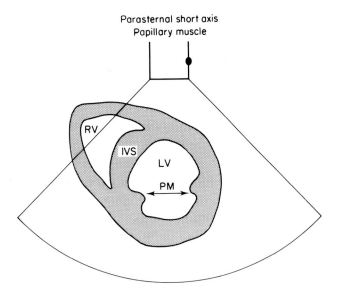

Figure 2.3d   Parasternal short axis plane at papillary muscle level.

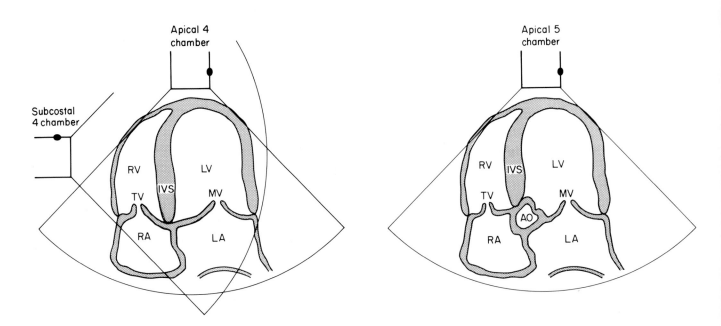

Figure 2.3e   Four chamber plane which can be visualized using both apical and subcostal transducer positions. By angling the transducer slightly anteriorly from the four chamber plane, the aortic valve and aortic root are included and this is called apical five chamber.

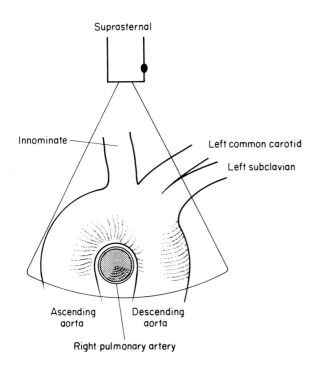

Figure 2.3f Suprasternal view of the aortic arch.

There will be occasions when a non-standard or modified view may be necessary to demonstrate particular anatomy or pathology. However, in order to develop a satisfactory scanning technique it is essential that the operator becomes completely fluent with the standard views. This will only be achieved after considerable practice so that the confidence to experiment with alternative views is realized. In this chapter the techniques for obtaining the standard views are described and also the most common scanning problems that are encountered.

All 2D transducers are provided with a distinguishing dot, mark, notch or button on one side near the transducer face. This dot defines the 2D scan plane. Structures which are imaged and positioned on this side of the transducer will conventionally be displayed on the right-hand side of the image seen on the screen. Some instruments also display a marker on the screen to remind the operator of the relationship between the transducer dot and the orientation of the displayed image. It is also usual to orient the image so that structures near the transducer are seen at the top of the screen, with the apex of the image pointing upwards. However, there are some pediatric echocardiography centers that prefer to display the image apex downwards for some particular views. This is so that the position of the displayed anatomy correlates better with the actual position in the body. This orientation of display may be confusing at first and is not illustrated in this book.

Parasternal long axis view

In many respects the parasternal long axis view of the heart provides the anchor point for many of the other imaging planes that we use. To obtain this view the transducer is placed on the left sternal edge in usually the third, fourth or fifth intercostal space. Occasionally, it may be necessary to use other intercostal spaces depending upon the position of the heart within the thoracic cavity and the availability of imaging windows. It is important to keep the transducer (despite which intercostal space is finally used) in toward the left sternal edge and not to wander out precordially unless absolutely necessary.

Depending upon the exact axis of the heart, the transducer dot should be pointing roughly toward the patient's right shoulder for the parasternal long axis view. As illustrated in Figure 2.3a, the scanning plane is correctly positioned when it transects the heart from the aortic root and through both the mitral valve leaflets and the main body of the left ventricle. The transducer will undoubtedly have to be moved in terms of position, angulation and rotation to obtain a satisfactory long axis image. These transducer movement terms are shown in Figure 2.4.

As mentioned previously, the transducer should be positioned on the left sternal edge. If possible, an intercostal space should be chosen so that the interventricular septum lies in a plane that is completely perpendicular to the transducer. If the aorta is positioned (on the image) in a higher position than the septum, a lower intercostal space should be used. Alternatively, if the aorta appears lower than the septum, a higher space is preferable. This point is demonstrated in Figure 2.5, and is important since it ensures that most of the anatomy lies perpendicular to the ultrasound

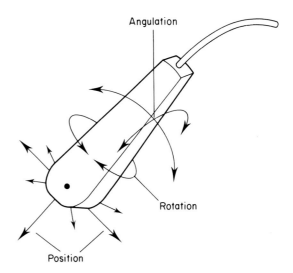

Figure 2.4 Terminology used to describe transducer movement on the chest, i.e. positional, rotational and angulation motion.

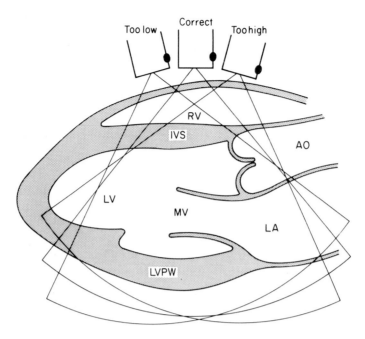

Figure 2.5 Parasternal long axis plane with the transducer placed correctly, too high and too low on the parasternal edge. With the transducer in the correct position, the aorta and interventricular septum should appear at the same height on both sides of the image plane.

pulses from the transducer and therefore stronger, more intense echoes will be generated. This increases the quality of both M-Mode and 2D images.

Angulation and rotation of the transducer have to be performed together and are dependent upon each other to obtain satisfactory images. The transducer should be angled so that the distance between the septum and posterior wall is at a maximum. This will ensure that the scanning plane will transect the left ventricle through its geometrical center and any measurements of cavity dimension will not be underestimated. Rotation of the transducer in both clockwise and counterclockwise directions should be performed so that the aorta and the left ventricle appear "open-ended". Due to the shape and length of the left ventricle, it is normally impossible to visualize the apex in a correctly oriented parasternal long axis image. Therefore if the ventricle appears closed off on the left-hand side of the image, this suggests that the rotation of the image plane is incorrect. The aorta is essentially a tube and so again it should not appear closed off on the right-hand side of the image. Both transducer rotation and angulation should be adjusted so the aortic root echoes appear as two parallel lines with maximum separation.

Parasternal long axis views of the right heart

With the transducer in the parasternal long axis position, it is normally possible to obtain two long axis views of the right heart. If the transducer is angled both medially and inferi-

orly, a long axis view of the right ventricular inflow tract and tricuspid valve is obtained, as shown in Figure 2.6a. Lateral and superior angulation of the transducer will produce an image of the long axis of the right ventricular outflow

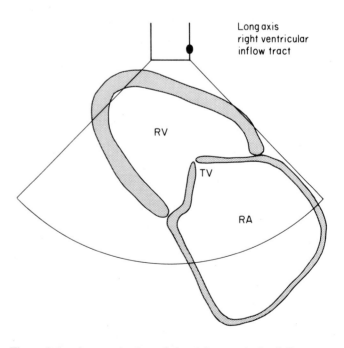

Figure 2.6a Long axis view of the right ventricular inflow tract with the transducer positioned in a parasternal position.

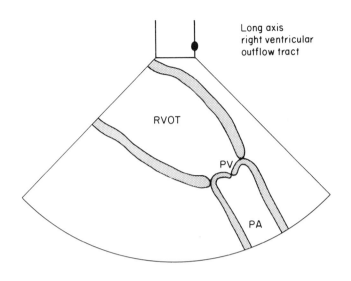

Figure 2.6b Long axis view of the right ventricular outflow tract.

tract, pulmonary valve and main pulmonary artery (see Figure 2.6b). These views are particularly useful when studying right heart pathology and should form part of the standard examination sequence whenever possible.

Parasternal short axis views

Parasternal short axis views are oriented at a 90° angle to the long axis plane. A clockwise rotation of the transducer is required so the dot is pointing roughly toward the left shoulder. There are three standard short axis views. These are obtained at the levels of the aortic valve, the mitral valve and finally the papillary muscles. These three views are illustrated in Figures 2.3b, c and d respectively.

With the dot pointing toward the left shoulder, the transducer is angled medially and superiorly to obtain a short axis image at aortic valve level. The exact angulation of the transducer is chosen so that the aortic valve leaflets are seen both centrally and symmetrically on the image plane. Transducer rotation is adjusted so that the aorta appears circular and both the right and left atria are visible. Since the aorta is a tube, a correctly oriented short axis image should demonstrate a circular rather than an ellipsoid shape. If the aorta appears as a vertically oriented ellipsoid then the transducer angulation is incorrect. A horizontally oriented ellipsoid suggests that adjustment to the transducer rotation is required.

If the transducer is now angled slightly inferiorly and laterally, a short axis view of the heart at mitral valve level will be obtained. At this point, the transducer will normally be oriented almost perpendicular to the chest wall. In this view both the anterior and posterior mitral valve leaflets should

be seen and will have a symmetrical appearance within the left ventricular cavity. This is shown in Figure 2.3c; it is important to note that the edges of the mitral leaflets on both the lateral and medial commissures are seen to the same extent. The left ventricular cavity itself should appear circular rather than ellipsoid. Minute adjustments of transducer angulation and rotation will be required to obtain correctly oriented views in much the same way as described for the aortic short axis view. Respiration will also have an effect on the position of the heart and, as mentioned previously, the patient may be required to hold their breath in expiration.

The short axis view of the left ventricle at papillary muscle level (Figure 2.3d) is obtained by further inferior and lateral transducer angulation. Again, the left ventricular cavity should appear circular with the tips of the two papillary muscles symmetrically positioned. Often the chordae tendineae are also included in this view. The right ventricular cavity may not be seen well in this plane since it is normally transected at the level of its apex.

Apical long axis view

The apical views tend to be the most difficult to acquire satisfactorily. This is undoubtedly because there is considerable variation in the position of the apex between patients. The most common scanning error is to place the transducer anteriorly, above the true apex, so that it is halfway between a parasternal and true apical position. With the transducer positioned incorrectly, as described, a foreshortened view of the ventricles will be obtained and the atria may not be satisfactorily imaged.

There are two easy ways to find the correct apical transducer position. If the apex can itself be palpated, then this location will invariably provide the most suitable transducer position. Alternatively, if the transducer is correctly positioned in a parasternal long axis view, it is possible to visualize the orientation of the scan plane in relation to the chest wall. The scan plane will point through the axis of the left ventricle toward the apex and the transducer should be moved over the chest, in the direction indicated, until a satisfactory apical view is obtained. At this point the distance between the transducer and mitral valve (the length of the ventricle) will be at a maximum. This is illustrated in Figure 2.3a.

If the transducer is maintained in the same plane as that used for the parasternal long axis view, then an apical long axis image is obtained and the dot will still be pointing roughly toward the patient's right shoulder. In this view, the apex of the left ventricle should be positioned exactly at the top of the image. Rotation and angulation of the transducer will be necessary to ensure that the aorta, mitral valve leaflets and left atrium are all included in the scan plane.

Apical four chamber view

The apical four chamber view is obtained using the same transducer position and angulation as above, but with approximately a 90° clockwise rotation so that the dot is pointing toward the left axilla. Figure 2.3e shows a correctly oriented four chamber view. The ventricular and atrial septum should be positioned centrally, down the image, with the right ventricle and atrium on the left side. It is useful to note that the tricuspid valve is inserted into the ventricular septum nearer the apex than the mitral valve. This provides a useful check on the position of the right ventricle, which is always attached to the tricuspid valve. If the atria are not included in the scan plane, then it is likely that the transducer should be positioned more posteriorly and/or angled anteriorly. Again, the distance between the transducer and the mitral valve should be at a maximum indicating that the scan plane is originating from the true anatomical apex. Transducer rotation is adjusted so that both the mitral and tricuspid valves are included within the scan planes and all four chambers are visible. Unless the cardiac anatomy is very unusual, the above technique will ensure a satisfactory four chamber image.

If the transducer is angled slightly anteriorly from the standard four chamber plane, a five chamber view is obtained. This view includes the aortic valve, aortic root and left ventricular outflow tract as shown in Figure 2.3e. It is rather inappropriately named since the aorta is not a chamber. However, this view is particularly useful for Doppler assessment of flow in the left ventricular outflow tract as described in Chaper 11.

Subcostal views

Subcostal views are often considered to be the most difficult to obtain and indeed they are certainly not possible in every patient. It is important to remember that, in this position, the transducer is further away from the heart than in other views. Therefore, only very small changes in transducer angulation are necessary to adjust the scan plane. The subcostal views are very useful for examining the right heart and in particular the interatrial septum. This very thin structure is normally oriented perpendicular to the scan plane in this view; there is therefore less chance of echo drop-out occurring. In examining patients with suspected atrial septal defects this is particularly relevant because apparent defects may occur in parasternal and apical views when the atrial septum runs parallel to the scan plane. In patients in whom it is impossible to obtain satisfactory parasternal views because of respiratory artefacts, the heart will often be lying low in the chest along the diaphragm. The subcostal views are very useful in these situations and therefore it is worthwhile becoming experienced in obtain-

ing them since, on occasions, they may be the only views of the heart available.

The patient should lie on their back in a semisupine position. Ideally, the subcostal area of the abdomen should be as relaxed as possible and it is usually useful if the legs are bent. The scan plane will be oriented so that it is running almost parallel with the rib cage. This is much easier to achieve if the length of the transducer is placed flat upon the abdomen so that it is pointing from almost the base of the sternum toward the left shoulder. The transducer should be held on top and while maintaining almost the same scan plane it should be pushed fairly firmly into the abdominal wall. If the patient inspires at this point, the subcostal access will invariably be increased as the lungs inflate, pushing the heart down toward the diaphragm and the rib cage outwards.

The four chamber view is the easiest subcostal image to obtain. The scan plane should transect the heart with virtually the same orientation as that achieved with the apical four chamber view. However, since the transducer position is now very different, the image will appear almost as an apical view rotated through approximately 90°, so that the septa now run across the image as shown in Figure 2.3e. The transducer dot should be pointing toward the patient's left side. Part of the liver will often be seen between the transducer and the heart and this is quite acceptable. As mentioned previously, small alterations in transducer position, rotation and angulation may be necessary to achieve a scan plane that includes all four chambers and the atrioventricular valves.

To obtain subcostal short axis views, the transducer dot should be pointing upwards (anteriorly). Again, these views should appear as parasternal short axis images seen from a different position. If the transducer is angled and pointed toward the neck, a short axis across the aorta, left atrium and pulmonary artery may be achieved. The latter structure is often seen particularly well in this view. With very small alterations in transducer rotation it is often possible to image the pulmonary veins entering the left atrium and the inferior vena cava and superior vena cava at their right atrial junctions.

By angling the transducer more toward the left shoulder and arm, short axis views of the ventricles at mitral valve and papillary muscle level may be obtained. Since access to the subcostal window is so limited, it is often necessary to accept images that are not optimally oriented in relation to the cardiac anatomy.

Suprasternal views

Suprasternal images are particularly useful for examining the aortic arch and the most superior aspects of the ascending and descending aorta. In order to obtain greatest access to the suprasternal window it is often necessary for the patient to lie flat on their back with a pillow under the shoulder blades so that the neck is stretched back. In addition, the head will usually need to be turned to one side. The transducer may be placed in the left, right or mid supraclavicular fossa, depending upon the exact position of the aortic arch. Some manufacturers supply angled transducers that are particularly suited to the suprasternal images and these are very useful in pediatric cases where access is limited.

If the aortic arch is normally positioned, the transducer dot should point roughly to the left side of the patient's neck so that the imaging plane will transect the long axis of the aorta over the arch. Since individual anatomy is so variable, transducer manipulation in terms of position, angulation and rotation will inevitably be necessary in order to achieve satisfactory images. A diagrammatic example of

a suprasternal image of the aortic arch is seen in Figure 2.3f. In pediatric and neonatal patients it is usually possible to visualize the ascending and descending aorta more extensively from this view than in adults. In addition, if the transducer is rotated so that the dot is pointing toward the right side of the neck, a suprasternal long axis image of the heart may be obtainable.

In adult patients it is unusual to be able to obtain all the 2D views described above in one individual. Indeed, in most adult patients, subcostal and suprasternal images are superfluous and do not contribute any additional information. However, since there are occasions where, because of pathology or limited scanning windows, these views are necessary, it is important that they are practised whenever possible. Representative, frozen 2D images of the standard views are shown in Figure 2.7 and may be compared with the diagrams in Figure 2.3.

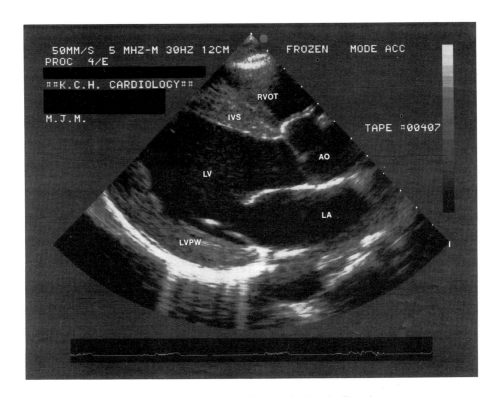

Figure 2.7a Parasternal long axis view in diastole.

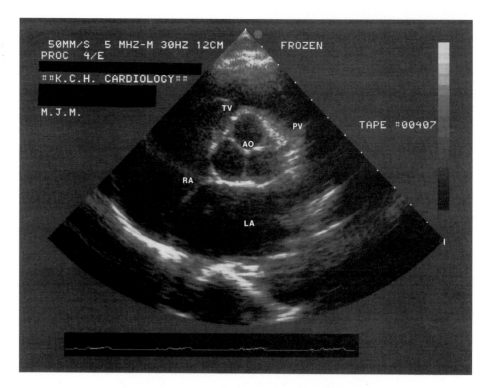

Figure 2.7b Parasternal short axis view in diastole.

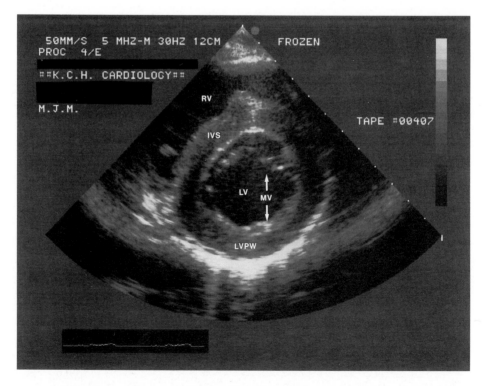

Figure 2.7c Parasternal short axis view at mitral valve level in diastole.

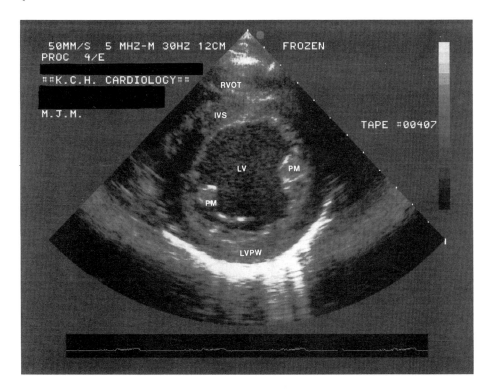

Figure 2.7d Parasternal short axis view at papillary muscle level in diastole.

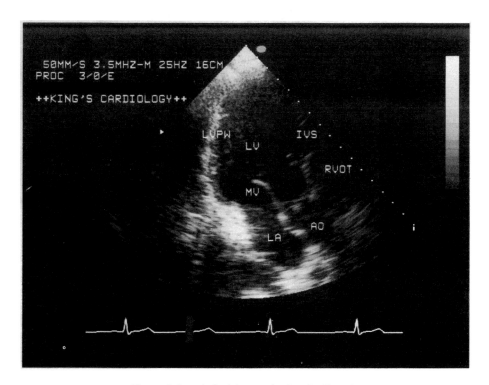

Figure 2.7e Apical long axis view in diastole.

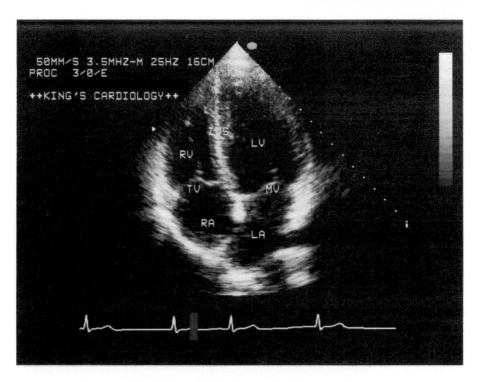

Figure 2.7f Apical four chamber view in systole.

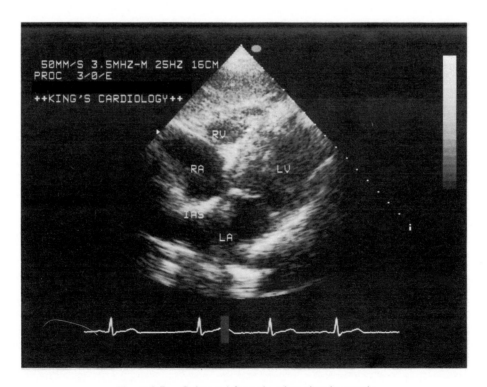

Figure 2.7g Subcostal four chamber view in systole

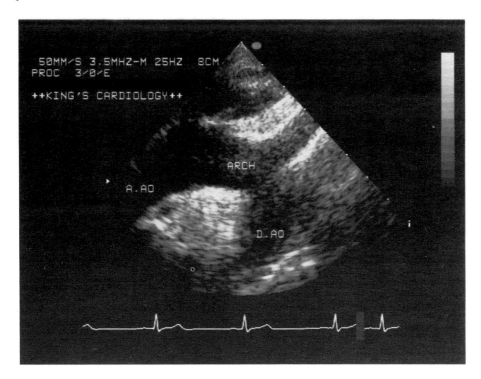

Figure 2.7h Suprasternal view demonstrating the long axis plane of the ascending aorta, aortic arch and descending aorta.

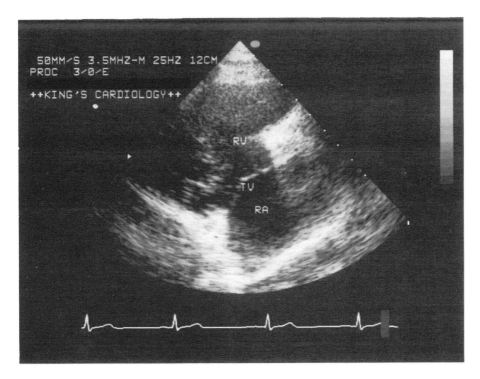

Figure 2.7i Parasternal long axis view of the right ventricular inflow tract in systole. This is obtained by tilting the transducer medially from the standard parasternal long axis view.

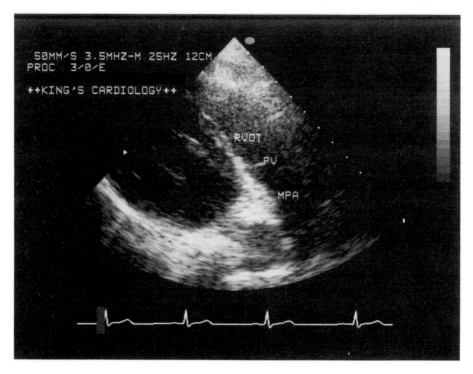

Figure 2.7j Parasternal long axis view of the right ventricular outflow tract showing the pulmonary valve and the main pulmonary artery. This is obtained by tilting the transducer laterally and superiorly from the standard parasternal long axis plane.

Standard M-Mode recording

Virtually all M-Mode recordings are obtained from the parasternal imaging window. Occasionally, subcostal M-Modes are used when parasternal views are not available.

As mentioned previously, it is important to ensure that, in order to achieve maximum recording quality, the M-Mode beam line crosses cardiac structures perpendicularly. In addition, if measurements of chamber size are made from an oblique M-Mode recording, the dimensions will be artefactually increased. Therefore, correctly oriented 2D views as described above should be used as a reference for selection of the M-Mode beam direction.

Standard M-Mode recordings normally would include the aortic root, aortic valve and left atrium as shown in Figure 2.8a, the right and left ventricle at mitral valve level (Figure 2.8b), the right and left ventricle at mitral chordal level (Figure 2.8c) and finally both the pulmonary and tricuspid valves (Figure 2.8d and e). It is possible to obtain most of these recordings using either parasternal long or short axis views as a reference. The alternative positions for the M-Mode left heart recordings are illustrated in Figure 2.9.

To make an aortic M-Mode recording, the beam position should be adjusted so that it travels across the aortic root (in a perpendicular fashion) at the level of the aortic

valve leaflets. The scan plane and beam position should be adjusted so that maximum separation of the aortic walls is achieved and additionally they should both have the same amplitude of motion. The posterior wall of the left atrium should always be included within the recording and the depth setting adjusted accordingly. The aortic valve leaflets should be seen; however, only the right and non-coronary leaflets are usually visible on M-Mode recordings. The instrument controls should be adjusted as suggested in Chapter 1 so that all the relevant structures are clearly seen but not artefactually thickened by excessive gain or transmit power.

When recording an M-Mode of the mitral valve, the beam position should be adjusted so that both leaflets are seen especially at their opening and closure points (C and D). It is a common mistake to record the mitral valve so that only the anterior leaflet is satisfactorily visualized. The posterior left ventricular wall and pericardium should be included in the recording. Adjustment of the near field gain controls may be necessary to demonstrate the right ventricular cavity (which should be echo free) and the anterior surface of the interventricular septum. Figure 2.8b is a demonstration of a technically good mitral valve level M-Mode recording.

The ventricular recording is achieved by positioning the beam just off the tips of the mitral valve leaflets at the level of the chordae tendineae so that the left ventricle is crossed at its maximum dimension. Again, the orienta-

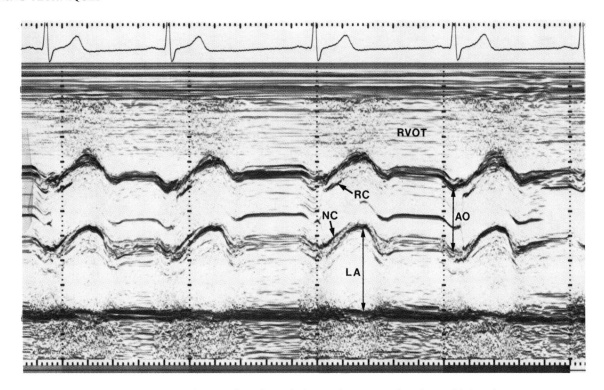

Figure 2.8a   M-Mode recording through the aortic root, aortic valve and left atrium.

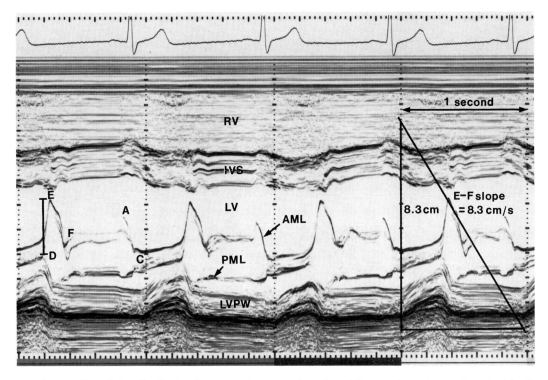

Figure 2.8b   M-Mode recording of the mitral valve demonstrating normal motion of the anterior and posterior mitral leaflets continuously throughout the cardiac cycle.

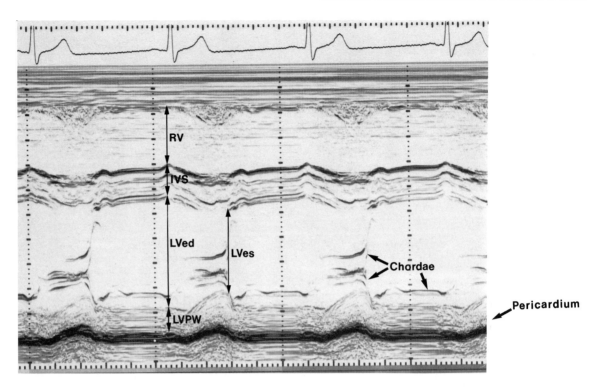

Figure 2.8c   M-Mode recording of the left ventricle just beyond the tips of the mitral valve leaflets at chordal level, demonstrating the right ventricle, the interventricular septum, the left ventricular cavity and left ventricular posterior wall. Recordings at this level are used for measuring left ventricular internal dimensions and myocardial wall thickness.

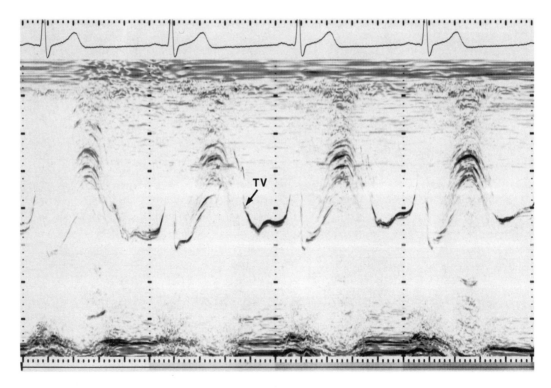

Figure 2.8d   M-Mode recording through the tricuspid valve. Because of the orientation of the M-Mode beam to the tricuspid leaflets, only one leaflet (usually the septal leaflet) is commonly recorded.

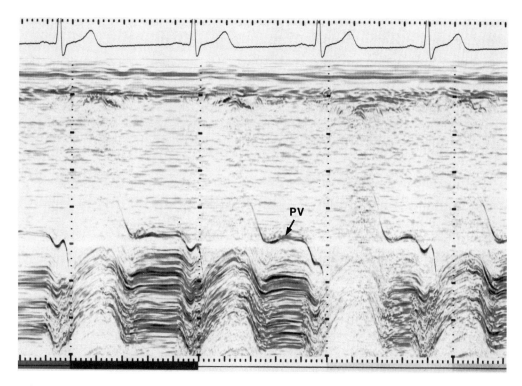

Figure 2.8e M-Mode recording through the right ventricular outflow tract, pulmonary valve and main pulmonary artery. One of the pulmonary valve leaflets is seen clearly during diastole. As the valve opens in systole it moves posteriorly and away from the transducer and is rarely recorded during systole except in patients with pulmonary stenosis.

tion of the beam should be perpendicular and this can be confirmed using the 2D image. An example is illustrated in Figure 2.8d and clearly demonstrates the anterior right ventricular wall, the right ventricular cavity, the interventricular septum (both right and left sides), the posterior left ventricular wall (especially the endocardium) and the posterior pericardium, which is normally a very dense echo.

It is easiest to record the tricuspid and pulmonary valves using a parasternal short axis 2D image at aortic level to orient the M-Mode beam. It may be necessary to angle the transducer slightly inferiorly and medially to visualize the tricuspid valve. An example of a tricuspid valve M-Mode and beam position is seen in Figure 2.8d. The normal motion pattern is similar to that of the anterior mitral valve leaflet. There are no additional relevant structures to be included in this recording.

To achieve a pulmonary valve recording, the beam position is lateral to the aorta as shown in Figure 2.9. If the pulmonary leaflets are not visible on the 2D image then the transducer should be moved down one interspace and angled in a more superior direction. In a significant proportion of patients it will still prove impossible to visualize the pulmonary valve since it is frequently obscured by lung tissue. A pulmonary valve M-Mode recording is illustrated in Figure 2.8e.

The normal orientation of the M-Mode beam to the right heart valves is such that only one of the valve leaflets is usually included in the recording. Therefore, more complete information about the appearance and motion of the leaflets is often obtainable from the real-time 2D images. However, recordings of these valves should be made (whenever possible) in every examination, if only to demonstrate that they have been studied.

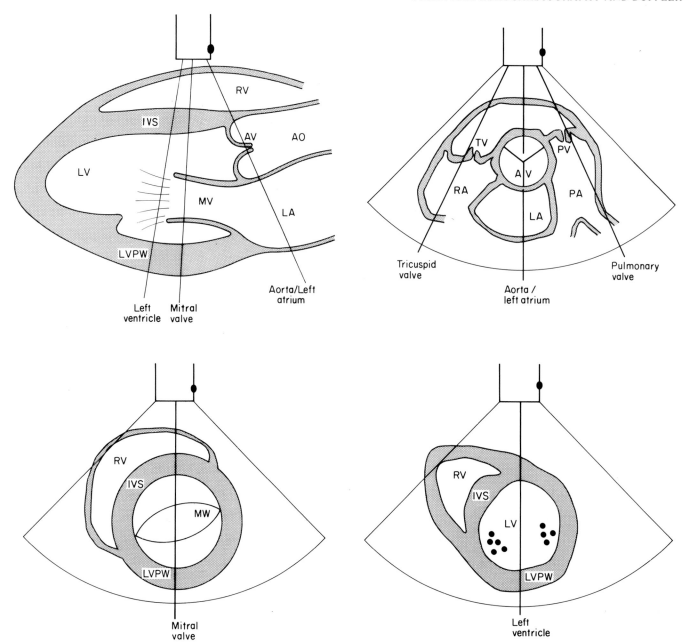

Figure 2.9   Diagrams showing M-Mode reference line positions derived from the parasternal long axis and parasternal short axis views.

It is important that the echo examination is always undertaken in a systematic and complete fashion. It may be necessary to make more extensive recordings of any relevant and obvious pathological abnormalities; however one should not be distracted away from examining the entire heart since other less prominent abnormalities may exist. Therefore an approach involving a systematic sequence of all views and recordings is a good habit.

CHAPTER 3

Analyzing the recording

This chapter discusses the basic techniques of making measurements (mainly from M-Mode recordings) and calculating some of the more commonly used parameters of left ventricular function. Some specific measurements, which would only be used in certain circumstances, are discussed at the appropriate point in the relevant chapters.

Most routine echo measurements are made from M-Mode recordings for several reasons. It is easy to make measurements at a specific point in the cardiac cycle, i.e. end-diastole and/or end-systole. Since cavity sizes and wall thicknesses alter so rapidly during the cycle, precise timing of measurements is important. In addition, the endocardial surfaces are usually defined better on M-Mode recordings than on 2D and this can make analysis easier.

Normal values for a variety of 2D measurements are now available. Providing the images are of sufficient quality and frozen at the appropriate point in the cardiac cycle there is no real reason why they should not be used.

One possible advantage of measuring from 2D images is that there is less possibility of geometrical distortion of the measurements. This would happen if the M-Mode beam was passing obliquely through a chamber and in this way creating artefactually increased dimensions. Therefore, the orientation of the M-Mode beam on the 2D image should always be checked before any recordings and measurements are made; this is illustrated in Figure 2.9. When it is not possible to obtain M-Mode recordings from the parasternal position, analysis of left ventricular dimensions etc. may be made from apical 2D images. However, if measurements are made which rely on the comparatively poor lateral resolution of 2D recordings, i.e. across the image plane, then caution needs to be exercised.

Timing of the points of measurement is usually done using the electrocardiogram for end-diastole and, if necessary, a carotid pulse trace recording to define end-systole. Diastolic measurements are made on the Q wave just at the beginning of the QRS complex, and systolic measurements are made at the point of aortic valve closure (the dichrotic notch). A more convenient, although less accurate, method to define end-systole is discussed under left ventricular measurements.

The apparent thickness of individual structures on both M-Mode and 2D recordings is dependent not only on the actual thickness of the structure itself but also on the length of the ultrasound pulse. If a long pulse length is being used the structure will appear to be thicker than it actually is. To eliminate the possibility of artefactually distorted measurements arising out of this problem, all measurements should be made from the leading edge of one echo to the leading edge of another. Thus, for example, when measuring the width of the aortic root as shown in Figure 2.8a, the distance between the anterior surface (leading edge) of the anterior wall and the anterior surface (leading edge) of the posterior wall is taken to be the dimension. The leading edges of these echoes are created only by the front of the ultrasound pulse and are therefore not dependent upon pulse length.

The easiest method of making measurements from hardcopy recordings is to use a pair of dividers and calculate the distance between two points utilizing the calibration scale on the recording. Unfortunately, this method is undoubtedly the least accurate and reproducible method. There are several commercial measuring systems available which use a digitizing tablet connected to a small computer. These systems are usually capable of making a large variety of echocardiographic measurements and incorporating some user selected text to produce a printed echo report. Measuring dimensions, areas and volumes from video images is a little more difficult. Fortunately, most modern ultrasound systems are equipped with a comprehensive analysis package which allows measurements to be made using a joystick or track-ball to control the position of the measuring cursor.

The aorta and left atrium (see Figure 2.8a)

The width of the aortic root is measured at the level of the aortic valve at end-diastole. As previously mentioned, ensure that the M-Mode beam is correctly geometrically aligned and use leading edge to leading edge dimensions.

The left atrial dimension is again recorded at aortic valve level. The maximum dimension which occurs at end-systole is measured. Indistinct and fuzzy echoes along the posterior left atrial wall can make identification of the true atrial wall difficult. This is best achieved by using the 2D image to decide which echo is the strongest and runs completely along the posterior aspect of the atrium. This structure may then usually be identified on the M-Mode recording.

The mitral valve (see Figure 2.8b)

Mitral valve measurements should be made only on recordings where both the anterior and posterior leaflets are seen continuously throughout diastole from their point of separation to coaptation at end-diastole. The mitral valve excursion (of the anterior leaflet) has been previously thought to represent the mobility of the valve. It is measured from the opening point of the leaflets (D point) to the point of maximum early diastolic motion of the anterior leaflet (E point).

The early diastolic closure slope of the mitral valve (E–F slope) is not commonly measured now. It was originally thought to be an indicator of the severity of mitral stenosis. However, the slope is clearly affected by many factors and is not reliable in this context. The time calibration markers are also needed to make this measurement, as shown in Figure 2.8b.

The left ventricle (see Figure 2.8c)

Measurements of the right and left ventricles, the septum and posterior left ventricular wall are usually made both at end-diastole and end-systole. The standard measurement points are illustrated.

The end-diastolic measurement points are readily identified from the electrocardiogram. While a carotid pulse trace recording may be used to identify end-systole, it is more convenient, albeit less precise, to define either the most posterior septal motion point or the most anterior motion point of the posterior left ventricular wall as end-systole. Providing that the motion of the septum or the posterior wall (whichever is used) is normal, either may be used to indicate end-systole since there will be little change in cardiac dimensions during the isovolumic phase which occurs between these points.

The right ventricle is usually crescent shaped and therefore its size on the M-Mode recording is dependent on the cardiac axis and also the position of the patient. For this reason, M-Mode measurements of right ventricular size are no longer considered to be very meaningful.

Identification of the true posterior left ventricular wall endocardial surface can frequently be complicated by the close proximity of chordal structures. These chordal echoes are usually less distinct, are not continuous for the entire cardiac cycle and do not move anteriorly in systole as fast as the true endocardial surface, which will have a steeper upward slope. These "rules" are often very helpful since it can be so easy to mistake the chordal echoes for the endocardium. The posterior wall epicardium is identified as the anterior surface of the dense posterior pericardial echo.

Left ventricular function and mass

One of the first described and simplest methods for calculating left ventricular volumes is the cubed technique. This method assumes that the left ventricle has an ellipsoid shape. The volume of an ellipsoid can be calculated by cubing the minor axis dimension. The minor axis of the left ventricle is in fact the same dimension that is measured from the standard M-Mode echo. Therefore, it is theoretically possible to calculate both the diastolic and systolic left ventricular volumes from an M-Mode recording by simply cubing the dimensions. This can be extended to allow both ejection fraction and stroke volume to be extrapolated by subtracting the systolic volume from the diastolic. If the stroke volume is multiplied by the heart rate, then cardiac output can also be calculated.

Left ventricular mass may be estimated in a similar way, by calculating the diastolic left ventricular volume and subtracting this from the entire volume of the left ventricle, septum and posterior wall (measuring from the anterior septal surface to the posterior wall epicardium). The resultant myocardial volume is then multiplied by the specific gravity of myocardium (1.04) to achieve a figure for left ventricular mass.

Unfortunately the above cubed methods, although very easy to apply, are subject to several possible errors. The largest of these errors is undoubtedly the assumption that the left ventricle is an ellipsoid shape. In normal healthy hearts this assumption may be almost valid. However, in patients with cardiac disease, especially those with myocardial pathology and/or left ventricular dilatation, the left ventricle will not be ellipsoid in shape. This factor should preclude the use of these techniques in just the kind of conditions where it might have proved most valuable. In addition, any small errors in measuring left ventricular dimensions will become much more significant when cubed and assume massive proportions if then multiplied by the heart rate! Despite the problems with these techniques, they are still occasionally used and quoted, especially for the calculation of left ventricular mass.

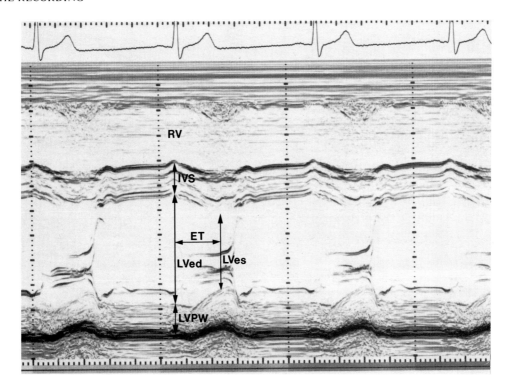

Figure 3.1 Example of various parameters of left ventricular function volume and mass which may be derived from left ventricular M-Mode recordings at mitral valve chordal level. For a full description of the relative merits and disadvantages of these techniques see the text.

$$\text{Fractional fiber shortening} = \frac{\text{LVed} - \text{LVes}}{\text{LVed}} \times 100\%$$

$$\text{Mean VCF} = \frac{\text{LVed} - \text{LVes}}{\text{LVed} \times \text{ET}} \quad s^{-1}$$

$$\text{Stroke volume} = (\text{LVed})^3 - (\text{LVes})^3 \quad ml^3$$

$$\text{LV mass} = (\text{LVed} + \text{IVS} + \text{LVPW})^3 - (\text{LVed})^3 \times 1.04 \quad g$$

There are two popular and simple M-Mode calculations for left ventricular function that do not use the cubed formula. One of these is called fractional fiber shortening and is essentially an echocardiographic equivalent of ejection fraction that is based upon left ventricular dimensions, as shown in Figure 3.1. The other frequently used calculation is of the mean circumferential fiber shortening velocity (mean VCF), which provides an estimate of left ventricular contractility, again based upon dimension measurements. However, this parameter does additionally use the ejection time (from a simultaneous carotid pulse trace) so that the rate of contraction can be calculated. A normal adult left ventricle has a mean VCF value of unity. The problem with all these M-Mode methods is that measurements of cavity dimensions at one single point are extrapolated to provide a figure representing the function or size of a complex three-dimensional structure.

In patients with abnormal left ventricular geometry, 2D echoes certainly have the potential to allow estimation of left ventricular volume more precisely. There have been a number of proposed methods utilizing combinations of various 2D imaging planes that have been shown to provide reasonably accurate volume calculations. To use any of these methods it is obviously essential that the 2D image quality is high so that the endocardium is well defined around the entire left ventricular wall.

The best currently available method for calculating volumes is a computer based technique called Simpson's Rule. This method is now built into most ultrasound image analysis systems and works by assuming that a three-dimensional chamber, such as the left ventricle, can be represented by many discs of varying diameters, rather like a stack of coins. Using a joystick or track-ball, the entire internal surface of the chamber is traced around. The long axis of the chamber

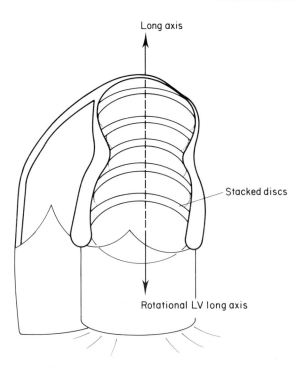

Figure 3.2 Diagram illustrating how Simpson's Rule may be used to calculate the volume of complex three-dimensional structures. The left ventricle, here shown represented in an apical four chamber plane, is divided by the computer system into a large number of discs of varying diameter. Only a few discs are shown in this diagram, but in reality all the discs would be touching each other and arranged around the central axis of the ventricle, which is also defined upon the image. The volume of the ventricle is calculated by summing the volume of all the individual discs.

is then defined and in the case of the left ventricle this is obviously from the apex to the mitral valve orifice at annular level. As shown in Figure 3.2, the computer will then calculate the chamber volume by stacking multiple discs of varying diameter (that will fit precisely across the width of the chamber) along the defined long axis line. By summing the volume of all the individual discs, an estimate of the total chamber volume can be achieved, even when the shape is irregular due to aneurysms etc.

However, it should be remembered that the computer is effectively rotating the two-dimensional chamber contour around its long axis to calculate a three-dimensional volume. It therefore assumes that the same chamber profile exists three-dimensionally, and this of course is rarely true. With more sophisticated analysis systems, two orthogonal imaging planes having the same long axis are traced into the computer. It is then possible to achieve a more accurate and reliable estimate of chamber volume, especially when the shape is very irregular. To calculate left ventricular volumes, the apical four chamber and/or apical long axis views would be used, since the entire cavity along its long axis can be visualized in these planes. These two views are orthogonal to one another and can be used for more precise volume estimation as described. To calculate any of the parameters of left ventricular function it is obviously necessary to measure both systolic and diastolic volumes.

CHAPTER 4

Mitral valve disease

The first pathology ever to be diagnosed by echocardiography was that of rheumatic mitral valve disease. Today, the assessment of conditions affecting the mitral valve remains an important application of the technique.

Rheumatic mitral stenosis

Rheumatic mitral valve disease progresses from commissural fusion of both the anterior and posterior mitral valve leaflets to infiltration of fibrous tissue which subsequently calcifies. This results in leaflet shrinkage and rigidity, with a narrowed mitral valve orifice producing hemodynamic obstruction to left ventricular filling. The distortion in mitral valve anatomy which this pathological process produces is so marked that it is easily detected by both M-Mode and 2D echo techniques.

Fibrosis and calcification are strong reflectors of ultrasound and produce dense, thickened echoes from a rheumatic valve. M-Mode examples of a normal and rheumatic valve are seen in Figures 4.1 and 4.2. The crys-

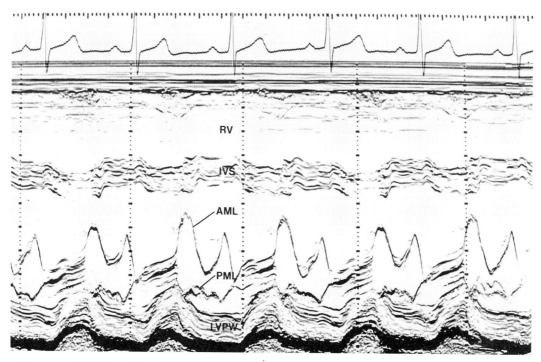

Figure 4.1 Normal M-Mode recording of the mitral valve. This demonstrates the classical M shape of the anterior leaflet with a mirror image W shape of the posterior leaflet during diastole. The leaflets are thin and mobile. The first diastolic peak is caused by early passive diastolic filling of the left ventricle through the mitral valve, and the late diastolic peak is caused by active filling as a result of atrial contraction.

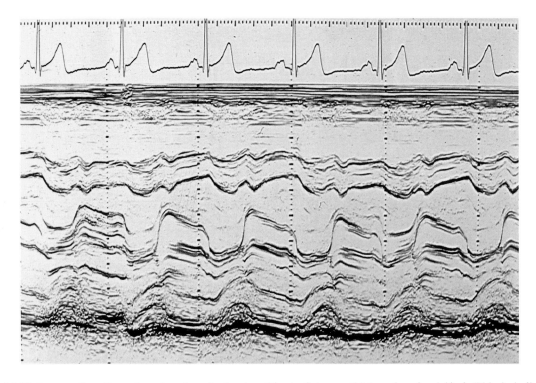

Figure 4.2a M-Mode recording through a stenotic mitral valve. The leaflets are thickened and calcified. This is indicated by echo reduplication. The mitral valve has lost the classic M shape of the anterior leaflet and the posterior leaflet moves anteriorly in diastole rather than posteriorly. The excursion of the anterior leaflet and the diastolic closing slope are reduced; in addition, the separation rate of the septum and the posterior left ventricular wall (during diastole) is slower, reflecting reduced left ventricular filling.

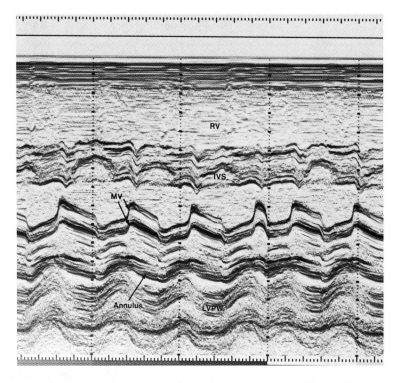

Figure 4.2b In this example the leaflets appear more extensively calcified with less mobility, and the posterior leaflet moves anteriorly in diastole. Posterior to the mitral leaflets a calcified mitral annulus is seen.

tals of calcium on the mitral valve cause the ultrasound pulses to reverberate and this results in multiple reduplicated echoes being detected by the echo equipment. These characteristic echoes can be seen on M-Mode recordings as parallel lines on the mitral valve leaflets. Echocardiography is almost certainly a more sensitive indicator of the presence of calcification than fluoroscopy. It is usually possible to appreciate different degrees of valvular calcification in the M-Mode by examining the thickness and extent of the reduplicated echoes. However the 2D echo is undoubtedly superior in this context because the overall distribution of calcification on the leaflets can be studied.

In patients with mitral stenosis, motion of the valve leaflets is abnormal and can be evaluated by both M-Mode and 2D echoes. Fusion of the commissures restricts the opening of the leaflets. Therefore the diastolic leaflet separation, as seen on the echo, is reduced. They remain at their maximum (although severely limited) separation during diastole. The biphasic filling of the ventricle is therefore usually lost except in very mild mitral stenosis.

In addition, the calcification and fibrosis reduce the mobility of the leaflets and this contributes to the loss of the normal M and W shape waveform patterns of the anterior and posterior leaflets respectively. As explained in the caption to Figure 4.1, the M and W mitral valve waveforms are due to the early and late diastolic filling phases of the ventricle. In patients with atrial fibrillation, the biphasic filling pattern will obviously not be present, and the mitral valve motion is abnormal irrespective of the presence of any mitral stenosis. In addition, loss of the M shape will occur in other conditions that are associated with low ventricular filling rates, hence it is not entirely specific to mitral stenosis. It is important to record the M-Mode of the mitral valve at the leaflet tips (where the posterior leaflet is also seen), since the leaflets are often more pliable and have greater mobility in their superior aspects.

Normally the posterior mitral leaflet moves posteriorly in diastole as shown in Figure 4.1. In mitral stenosis it is either immobile, or moves slightly anteriorly, as shown in Figure 4.2. This is due both to the calcification/fibrosis and to the anterior force exerted upon it by the anterior leaflet through the fused commissures. In patients with very mild rheumatic mitral valve disease it is often this restriction in the motion of the posterior leaflet that is the only indicator of valve pathology.

Measurement of the mitral valve excursion (to assess valve mobility) and the early diastolic (E–F) closure slope of the mitral valve is possible from M-Mode recordings. However, as previously mentioned, abnormalities of these parameters are not specific for mitral stenosis and, in addition, the severity of the disease is better judged from 2D echo.

The M-Mode appearances of a stenotic mitral valve therefore have three characteristic features: calcification and fibrosis of the leaflets denoted by thickened, dense and reduplicated echoes, loss of the M waveform shape of the anterior leaflet with reduction in the (E–F) closure slope, and immobility or slight diastolic anterior motion of the posterior leaflet.

The 2D echo appearances of mitral stenosis are, in their own way, just as characteristic as the M-Mode appearances and convey important additional information. There is obviously a better overall appreciation of the mobility of the leaflets and the distribution of calcification. These are important factors in considering the suitability of a mitral valve for valvotomy or valvuloplasty as opposed to valve replacement. Good leaflet mobility and lack of significant calcification are prerequisites of this type of procedure and should always be considered in any echo evaluation of a stenotic mitral valve.

Calcification in the mitral valve annulus, as distinct from the leaflets, can also be seen on the echo, as shown in Figure 4.3, and is additional relevant information.

In the absence of any other pathology that would cause reduced transvalvar flow, a normal mitral valve has leaflets that open freely and widely and this can be easily seen on the moving, real-time 2D images. A normal frozen image example is seen in Figure 2.7a and this can be compared with Figure 4.4, which demonstrates the classical 2D appearances of mitral stenosis. A stenotic mitral valve has a domed diastolic appearance. This can be seen using either the long axis or apical four chamber image planes. The main body of the valve separates more widely than the leaflet edges and the fused commissures. This is due to the pressure of blood building up behind the leaflets as it tries to pass through the narrowed orifice. It is rather analogous to the bulging of a yacht sail with the pressure of the wind behind it. The sudden doming of the valve at the beginning of diastole can be seen very clearly on real-time images and coincides with the auscultatory mitral opening snap. Another example of mitral valve doming is seen in Figure 4.5.

In heavily calcified mitral valves with poor mobility it may be difficult to appreciate the valve actually opening and doming since the restriction in valve motion is as much due to calcification as commissural fusion. However, in more pliable valves, the main body of the leaflets move well with only the tips tethered by commissural fusion and chordal shortening. Using parasternal short axis images, the commissural fusion at the medial and lateral edges of the leaflet tips can be seen in that the anterior and posterior leaflets remain fixed together at those points during the entire cardiac cycle (Figure 4.6).

Although both the M-Mode and 2D appearances of rheumatic mitral valve disease have a high diagnostic sensitivity, it is only using 2D echo that it is possible to assess the severity of any stenosis. This is accomplished by evaluation of the mitral valve orifice area, which obviously requires imaging in both the lateral and axial planes. The complete shape and area of the orifice can then be appreciated.

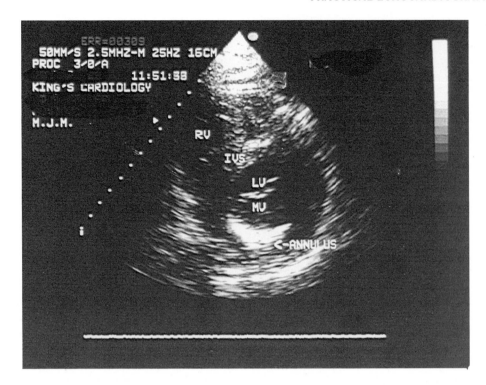

Figure 4.3 Parasternal short axis view at mitral valve level in a patient with a calcified mitral valve annulus. The very bright crescent-shaped echoes originating from the posterior annulus are clearly seen and are separate from the mitral valve leaflet echoes which are positioned more anteriorly.

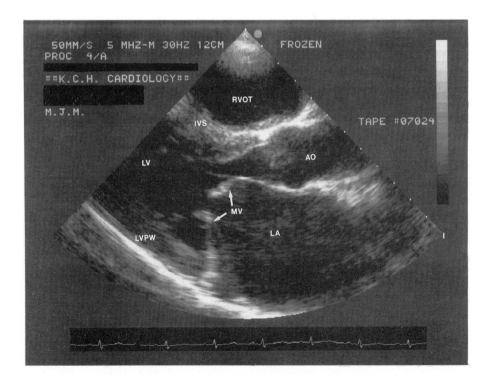

Figure 4.4 Parasternal long axis view in diastole in a patient with rheumatic mitral stenosis. The left atrium is dilated and there is classical doming of the anterior and posterior mitral valve leaflets, leaving a narrowed orifice for blood to flow through the valve into the left ventricle.

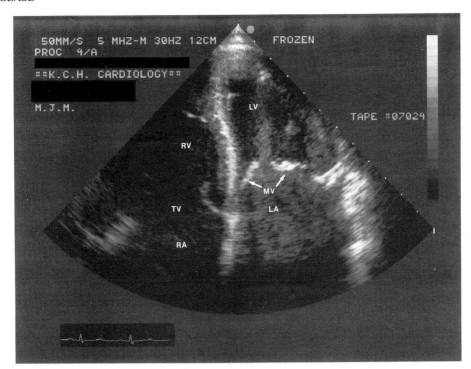

Figure 4.5 Apical four chamber view in diastole showing doming of both the anterior and posterior mitral valve leaflets in a patient with mitral valve stenosis. In addition a cloud of echoes (spontaneous echo contrast) can be seen entering the left ventricle through the mitral valve orifice. This phenomenon occurs as a result of red blood cell aggregation within the left atrium where some stagnation of blood is undoubtedly occurring. Occasionally these red blood cell aggregates become large enough to reflect ultrasound and cause apparent opacification of blood flow. Within the left ventricular cavity these aggregates disperse and therefore the spontaneous contrast disappears. Studies have demonstrated that this finding is associated with a higher than normal incidence of embolic events.

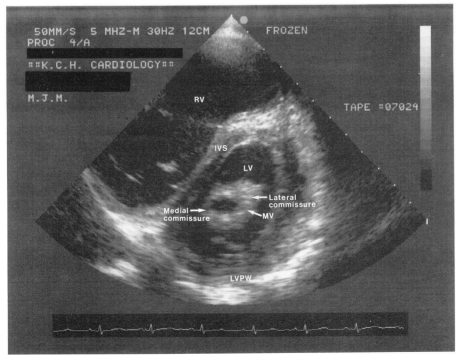

Figure 4.6 Parasternal short axis view of the mitral valve demonstrating calcified and thickened leaflets in a patient with mitral stenosis. The leaflets are fused together at both the lateral and medial commissures and the resultant valve area is markedly reduced. In addition, this patient has severe pulmonary hypertension secondary to the mitral valve disease and consequently the right ventricle is grossly dilated and is compressing the left ventricle, which now has a D shape (in short axis) rather than the normal circular short axis configuration.

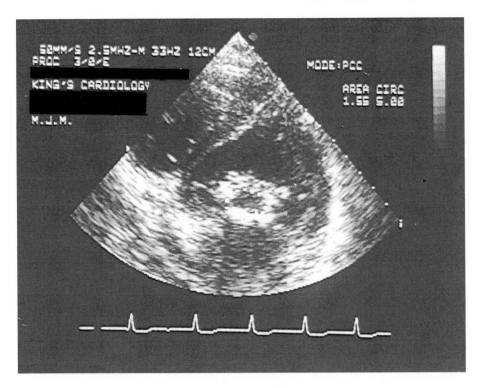

Figure 4.7 Parasternal short axis view of the mitral valve in a patient with mitral stenosis and reduced mitral valve area. The internal edges of the mitral valve orifice (at the leaflet tips) have been planimetered using an on-line image analysis system. The mitral valve area is calculated at 1.5 cm², which would suggest mild stenosis.

As shown in Figure 2.7c, the mitral valve normally opens so wide (during the filling phases) that when the orifice is viewed in short axis it occupies most of the left ventricular cavity in that plane. Hence it is often described as having a "fish-mouth" appearance. In mitral stenosis the reduced orifice size is usually easily seen and does not change appreciably during diastole. In normal adults, the mitral valve area is approximately between 3 and 5 cm²; in severe stenosis it is less than 1 cm², in moderate stenosis between 1 and 1.5 cm² and in mild cases greater than 1.5 cm². An example is illustrated in the short axis 2D echo seen in Figure 4.7.

Correct short axis imaging of the mitral valve orifice requires great care. The complex funnel shape of the stenotic valve means that it is possible to overestimate the valve area by imaging obliquely or too near the aorta. However by using the following approach these problems may be minimized. Start with a correctly aligned parasternal long axis view, using the appropriate intercostal space (as described in Chapter 2) and with the mitral valve leaflet tips positioned exactly in the center of the image (the posterior leaflet will usually appear almost vertical). Without changing the position or angulation of the transducer, rotate it through 90° into the short axis plane. In theory, you should now have a mitral short axis at the leaflet tips. Angle the transducer slightly toward the apex so that the scan plane just leaves the mitral leaflets. Then angle back up again toward the

valve until the first point when both the anterior and posterior leaflets (with the commissures) can be seen. The image can then be frozen during diastole for mitral valve area measurement.

With modern echocardiographic analysis systems it is possible to trace around the internal edge of the orifice with a light pen or electronic calipers and planimeter the mitral valve area. Measurements of mitral valve area obtained by this technique appear to correlate very well with both surgical and post-mortem findings and allow separation of mitral stenosis into mild, moderate and severe categories. Mitral valve area is obviously a more accurate reflection of stenosis severity than the pressure gradient (obtained by catheterization) because it is independent of transvalvar flow, i.e. cardiac output. In addition, there are many problems with the measurement of mitral valve area using invasive cardiac catheterization techniques. It is likely that echocardiography reflects more accurately the anatomical and functional state of the mitral valve than any other diagnostic tool.

The increase in left atrial pressure secondary to mitral stenosis causes dilatation of the left atrial cavity and this should always be measured on the echo. (The 2D echo in Figure 4.5 also shows a dilated left atrium.) The extent of left atrial enlargement is limited by atrial wall rigidity but is also a reflection of the severity and duration of the steno-

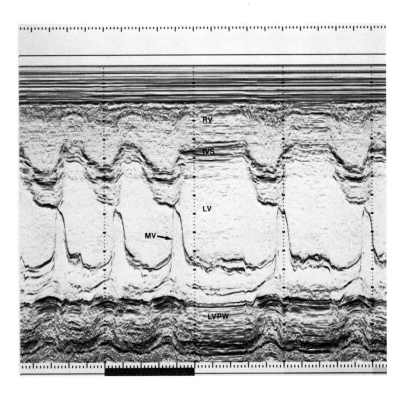

Figure 4.8 M-Mode recording of the left ventricle in a patient with severe mitral regurgitation. Left ventricular dimensions are increased and there is exaggerated, hyperdynamic motion of the septum and posterior ventricular wall. This reflects increased left ventricular stroke volume due to blood leaking back through the mitral valve into the left atrium. In addition, the mitral valve excursion is increased.

sis. Thrombus can collect in the dilated left atrium and may often be seen on the 2D echo (see Chapter 9). It is important to check for thrombus because, if present, it may be an indication for early anticoagulation. Unfortunately the left atrial appendage is a common site for thrombus to accumulate and this is not seen well on any echo view. Indistinct, fuzzy echoes in the region of the posterior left atrial wall are common and do not necessarily indicate thrombus. This complicates the diagnosis of thrombus further. However, the incidence of false positives may be reduced by ensuring that the suspected thrombus is visualized in at least two separate views.

Raised left atrial pressure will also have an effect upon right heart hemodynamics, causing pulmonary hypertension, right ventricular hypertrophy and tricuspid incompetence. Mitral stenosis and these other conditions can also be evaluated to a greater or lesser extent by Doppler echocardiography and are discussed in more detail in Chapter 11.

Mitral regurgitation

Conventional echocardiography only provides us with indirect evidence of the presence of mitral regurgitation. The stethoscope is a more convenient and certainly more cost-effective diagnostic tool in this context!

Although echocardiography is relatively insensitive in the diagnosis of a mitral valve leak, it does play a useful role in determining the pathogenesis and hemodynamic consequences. Both of these factors are prognostically important.

The raised mitral valve flow may cause increased diastolic excursion of the leaflets (<2 cm). However, this is not a specific indicator. In addition, the leaflet fibrosis and restriction that occurs in rheumatic mitral valve disease will decrease the leaflet excursion as described in the previous section. Unfortunately the resolution of current equipment does not usually facilitate direct imaging of the systolic leaflet separation.

The indirect indicators of regurgitation can be seen on both M-Mode and 2D echoes. These are primarily volume overload of both the left atrium and the left ventricle with consequent dilatation. The left ventricular stroke volume will be increased, with exaggerated motion of both the ventricular septum and the posterior left ventricular wall, as seen in Figure 4.8. In severe regurgitation the aortic ejection time will be reduced and this can be seen as a gradual systolic closure of the aortic valve on M-Mode recordings.

In patients with mitral stenosis, the only clue to coexistent regurgitation will be that of left ventricular dilatation.

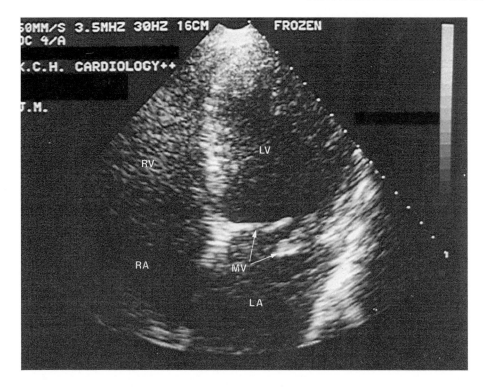

Figure 4.9 Apical four chamber view in a patient with ruptured chordae on the posterior mitral valve leaflet. In this systolic frame, part of the mitral valve apparatus and the chordae can be seen prolapsing behind the anterior leaflet into the left atrium.

Although the left atrium is dilated in mitral stenosis, the left ventricle is usually small if there is no regurgitation. If regurgitation is the main lesion in a patient with mitral disease then restriction of the posterior leaflet may be the only rheumatic change.

Other etiologies of regurgitation that can be detected by echo include mitral valve prolapse, ruptured chordae, papillary muscle dysfunction and endocarditis. An example of ruptured chordae on the posterior leaflet is seen in Figure 4.9. In this systolic image the chordae can be seen prolapsing back into the left atrium.

Both M-Mode and 2D techniques will provide an assessment of left ventricular function. This is very useful in any patient with valvular heart disease since poor function is likely to preclude a surgical management approach. It is therefore helpful to include an assessment of left ventricular function in the echo report.

Doppler techniques (Chapter 11) are extremely sensitive in the detection of mitral regurgitation and can also be used to quantify the severity of the leak. The technique is also very precise in measuring the severity of mitral stenosis and complements the anatomical and functional information available from standard echo.

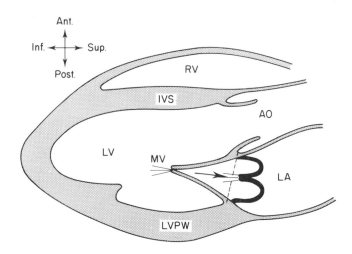

Figure 4.10 Diagrammatic representation of the parasternal long axis image in systole showing both the normal and prolapsed positions (in black) of the mitral valve leaflets. This diagram demonstrates severe prolapse of both the anterior and the posterior mitral valve leaflets; however, a systolic image would be considered diagnostic if either leaflet moved beyond the atrioventricular plane illustrated with a dotted line.

Mitral valve prolapse

Echocardiographic studies have suggested that the incidence of mitral valve prolapse may be as high as 20% in young females, whereas various post-mortem studies report incidences of between 3 and 5% in females and between 0.5 and 1% in males. These disparities almost certainly reflect the absence of an accurate gold standard for the diagnosis of prolapse. Since the mitral valve prolapse syndrome has been associated with other clinical findings, including cerebral ischemic events and susceptibility to bacterial endocarditis, the establishment of a definitive diagnosis in an individual patient is very important.

In this condition the pathological abnormalities are increased surface area of the mitral valve leaflets and lengthened chordae. Myxomatous or collagen degeneration of the valve tissue is also frequently present.

During ventricular systole the high left ventricular pressure causes the redundant valve tissue to invaginate into the left atrium. This is the origin of the late systolic murmur and/or systolic click found in this condition. Prolapse may affect either or both mitral valve leaflets and is very commonly seen in the medial scallop of the posterior leaflet.

The prolapsing motion of the valve leaflets can usually be appreciated with both M-Mode and 2D echocardiography. A 2D recording is considered compatible with prolapse if the valve tissue is seen to move beyond the atrioventricular plane into the the left atrium during systole. Ideally, this should not only be seen in the long axis view, shown diagrammatically in Figure 4.10, but also in the apical four chamber view, as illustrated in Figure 4.11. It is often helpful to either imagine or actually draw a line from one side of the valve annulus to the other. If either one or both of the leaflets move beyond that line during mid and/or late systole then prolapse must be suspected. The apical four chamber view is slightly less specific for the diagnosis of prolapse than the long axis imaging planes.

Figure 4.12 is a normal, long axis, systolic image and should be compared with Figure 4.13, which is recorded from a patient with mitral valve prolapse involving mainly the posterior leaflet. Here the buckled posterior leaflet (arrowed) can be seen protruding into the left atrium. This is often easier to appreciate in real time. As the valve leaflets move in a superior plane into the atrium there is usually also a small posterior motion component. It is that posterior motion that can be seen on the M-Mode echo.

In the M-Mode recordings of Figures 4.14 and 4.15, there is an abrupt posterior motion of part of the mitral valve

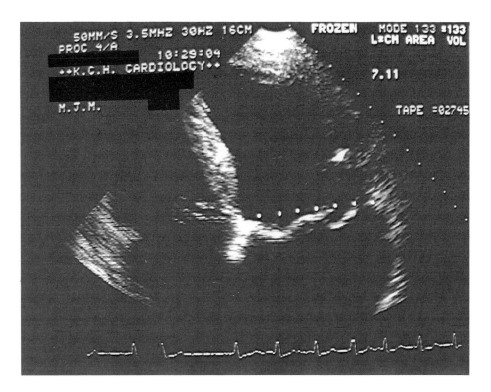

Figure 4.11 Systolic apical four chamber view in a patient with prolapse of both the anterior and posterior mitral valve leaflets. A dotted line representing the atrioventricular plane is shown and connects the hinge points of both the leaflets respectively. During systole, both leaflets move beyond this plane into the left atrium. It should be noted that the apical four chamber plane is rather less specific than either of the long axis planes for the diagnosis of prolapse.

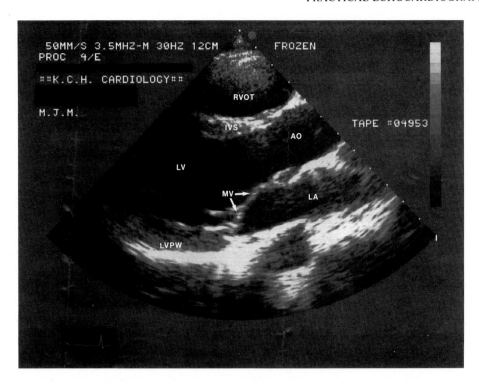

Figure 4.12 Parasternal long axis systolic image in a normal patient. The systolic position of the anterior and posterior mitral valve leaflets is in front of an imaginary line drawn across the atrioventricular plane.

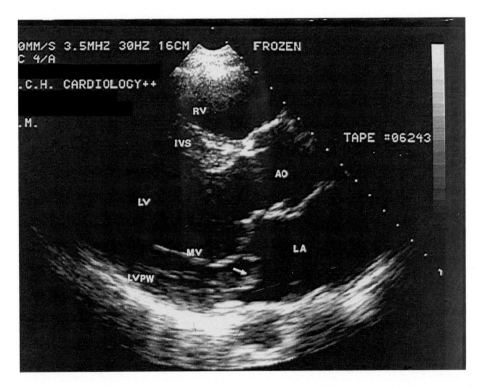

Figure 4.13   In this parasternal long axis image the posterior leaflet can be seen buckling and prolapsing (arrowed) into the left atrium.

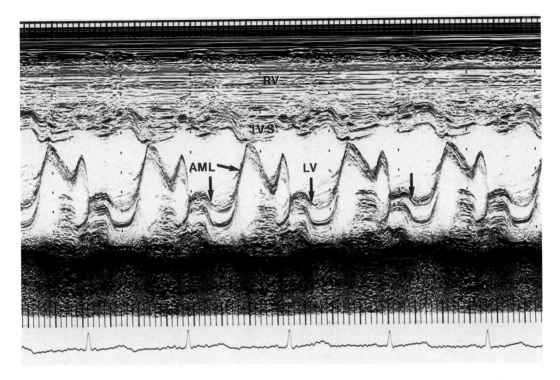

Figure 4.14 M-Mode recording of late systolic mitral valve prolapse. In mid systole (arrowed) the entire mitral valve apparatus moves posteriorly as the leaflets buckle into the left atrium.

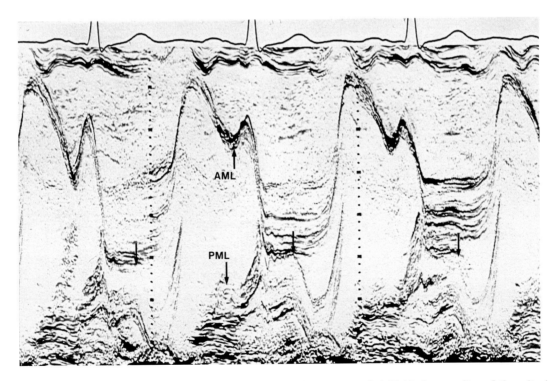

Figure 4.15 Another example of late systolic mitral valve prolapse, using an expanded M-Mode recording of the mitral valve. In this example only part of the mitral valve apparatus moves posteriorly, while the remaining valve and chordal structures exhibit normal systolic motion.

echoes. This motion can be seen to start in mid to late systole. The M-Mode is essentially a recording of depth against time; therefore it is easy to determine if the prolapse is of the late or holosystolic type. Figures 4.14 and 4.15 illustrate the former. If the posterior hammocking of the mitral valve echoes had started at the beginning of systole this would have been indicative of holosystolic or pansystolic prolapse, as shown in Figure 4.16.

Both the M-Mode and 2D techniques are entirely complementary in the evaluation of patients with suspected mitral valve prolapse. The M-Mode can only appreciate axial motion and is therefore dependent upon detecting any posterior movement in the prolapsing valve. It therefore has a lower sensitivity and specificity than the 2D echo, where the spatial orientation of the valve and its relationship to the atrioventricular ring may be seen. In addition, false positive and false negative M-Mode recordings can arise by too posterior or superior positioning of the transducer respectively. Furthermore, a very early systolic slight (<0.5 cm) posterior motion of the leaflets on the M-Mode is normal and is due to movement of the entire valve annulus rather than prolapse. Thus, while the M-Mode is not very useful in diagnosing or excluding prolapse, it does allow differentiation between holosystolic and late systolic prolapse which can be difficult to determine on the 2D echo.

Some degree of mitral regurgitation is frequently coexistent with prolapse and this may be evaluated with Doppler techniques as previously mentioned.

Although mitral prolapse is usually benign, there are a large number of patients who have significant clinical problems and there is a proliferation of echocardiographic literature on the subject. This undoubtedly reflects the uncertainty of the clinical significance of echo abnormalities that have been described in the condition. Nevertheless, the diagnosis of mitral prolapse remains an important application of echocardiography and it is probably the most widely used and most accurate method of diagnosis.

Prosthetic mitral valves

The assessment of prosthetic valve function is relatively difficult using conventional echocardiography and usually more meaningful information is obtainable from Doppler, as described in Chapter 11. In this section some general guidelines on the kind of information that can be derived using conventional echo are given.

Tissue bioprosthetic valves are slightly easier to evaluate than the other types of metal and/or plastic prostheses. This is because it is often possible to directly visualize the valve leaflets which are most commonly made of porcine valve or pericardial tissue. The leaflets are usually supported by three stents attached to the valve sewing ring. These structures are made of metal and are therefore strongly echo reflectant; they may obscure visualization of the leaflet thickness and motion in some views. In Figure 4.17 a normal mitral heterograft prosthesis (made from porcine aortic valve) is seen. The valve leaflets are thin and mobile and have the expected appearance of a normal aortic valve suspended between the strongly reflectant stents. Obstruction of the valve by thrombus or leaflet fibrosis/calcification is easier to appreciate using 2D echo because of the multiple views available and also the spatial orientation which the technique affords.

Nonbioprosthetic valves are very echo reflectant and it can be extremely difficult to appreciate the anatomy and mobility of the ball or disc, even using 2D echo. If there is clinical evidence of valve obstruction and reduced or severely limited mobility of the valve mechanism is seen, then the echo may be considered compatible with obstruction. The mobility of the valve is usually best appreciated using an apical imaging window as shown in Figure 4.18. However, since there can be considerable variability in the echo appearance of nonbioprosthetic valves, it is extremely difficult to be certain about any deterioration in valve function without a baseline echo for comparison. Therefore, if

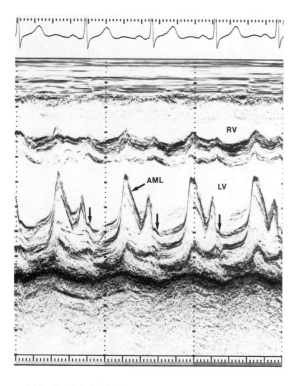

Figure 4.16 In this M-Mode recording the mitral valve prolapse is described as holosystolic or pansystolic. Prolapsing motion of the leaflets commences at the start of systole (arrowed) and continues throughout. Note that a small initial posterior motion of the mitral valve apparatus at the beginning of systole is quite common. However, in normal patients this does not continue throughout systole.

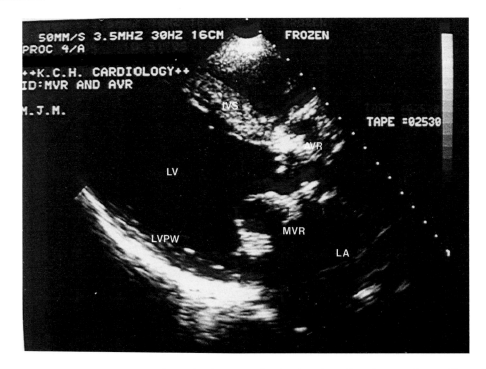

Figure 4.17a Parasternal long axis view in a patient with heterograft mitral and aortic valve prostheses. Since these are both tissue prostheses, only the stents supporting the valve leaflets are clearly seen in these still images. When the leaflets become abnormally thick and calcified they are more readily appreciated.

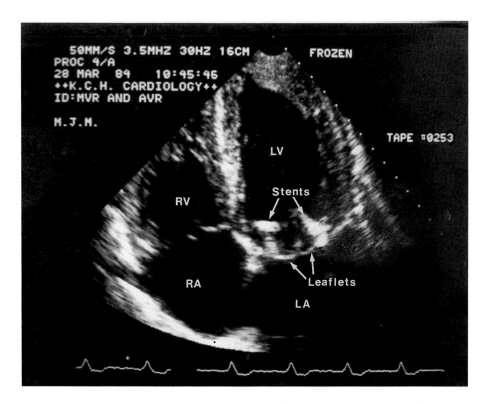

Figure 4.17b When the mitral valve prosthesis is visualized in this apical four chamber view, the leaflets are oriented perpendicular to the transducer and are therefore better appreciated as they sit in systole, suspended between the prosthetic stents.

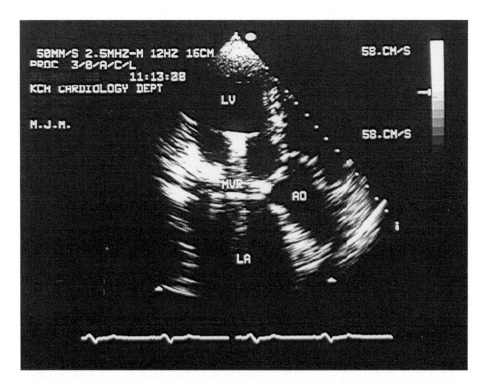

Figure 4.18 Apical long axis view in a patient with a Starr Edwards mitral valve prosthesis. The metallic cage and valve apparatus can be seen protruding into the left ventricle and in moving real-time images the motion of the occluder can be appreciated.

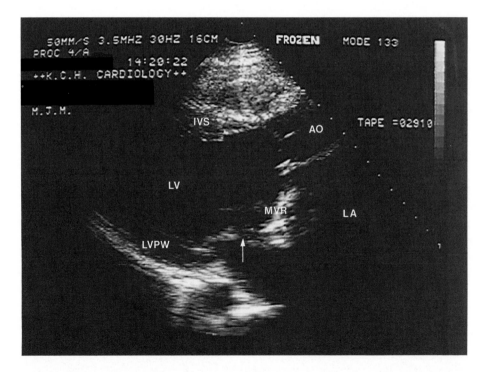

Figure 4.19 Parasternal long axis view in a patient with severe prosthetic valve dehiscence. The posterior aspect of the valve sewing ring has become completely separated from the mitral annulus (arrowed). During systole the whole prosthesis prolapsed back into the left atrium, hanging from its anterior attachment.

prosthetic valve function has to be evaluated without the additional hemodynamic information available from Doppler, then it may be useful to record baseline echoes on all patients early after valve replacement so that any deterioration is easier to detect.

Prosthetic valve regurgitation may be inferred using the same criteria described for native valves. In addition, if the valve leak is paraprosthetic then it is often possible to visualize excessive motion of part of the sewing ring at the point of valve dehiscence. This may require very careful examination using parasternal long axis and also apical views. An example of severe valve dehiscence that was evident even on a frozen 2D image can be seen in Figure 4.19.

The echo appearances of the mitral valve were first described by Edler in 1956. It is certainly the easiest of all the cardiac valves to image in most cases and even mild abnormalities can produce striking echocardiographic changes. It is now possible to avoid cardiac catheterization in many patients with uncomplicated mitral valve disease.

CHAPTER 5

Aortic valve disease

This chapter discusses the assessment of both acquired and congenital aortic valve disease using conventional echocardiography. The first echocardiographic description of the aortic valve was by Edler in 1961 using M-Mode. With the subsequent advent of 2D echo and Doppler, precise anatomic and hemodynamic data relating to aortic valve function can be obtained on virtually all patients. No other diagnostic technique, invasive or non-invasive, can compete with echocardiography. The technique is therefore now a mandatory examination in any patient suspected of having any form of aortic valve or root pathology.

Congenital aortic valve disease

Isolated aortic valve disease is almost always congenital in origin and therefore usually secondary to a bicuspid valve. This is a mild defect, present in about 1% of the population.

In the young patient without significant aortic valve thickening and calcification it is normally possible to directly visualize the anatomy of the valve leaflets with 2D echo. Using the short axis image plane, as shown in Figures 5.1, 5.2 and 5.3, the configuration of the valve leaflets can be

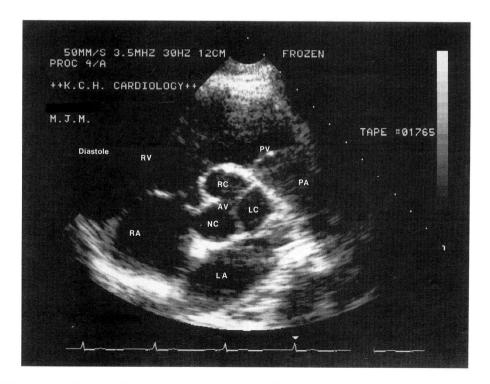

Figure 5.1 Diastolic parasternal short axis view of the aortic valve. The three valve leaflets can be clearly seen and the normal Y configuration of the commissures in diastole is evident.

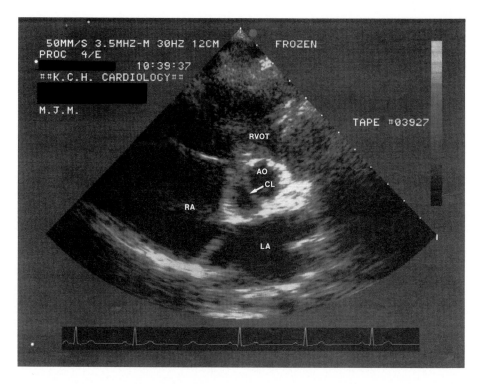

Figure 5.2 Aortic valve short axis view in a patient with a bicuspid aortic valve demonstrating a single closure line.

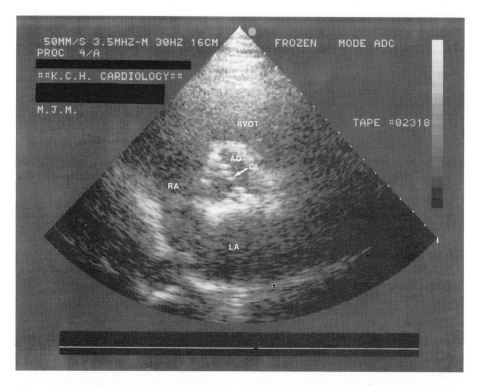

Figure 5.3 This example is similar to Figure 5.2. However, in this case the leaflets have begun to calcify and fibrose and therefore the closure line is more evident. This valve was moderately stenotic with a peak aortic pressure gradient of 60 mmHg.

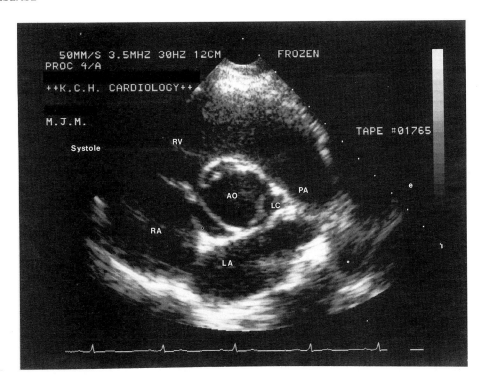

Figure 5.4 Short axis view of the aortic valve in systole demonstrating the normal triangular shape of the aortic valve orifice.

seen. It is possible to differentiate between a bicuspid and a normal valve. The latter has a Y shape in diastole, this pattern representing the diastolic closure line of the leaflet commissures. In a bicuspid valve a single closure line, with variable orientation, is usually seen. However, in some functionally bicuspid aortic valves two of the three cusps may be simply joined together and the fused raphe will remain echo reflective. This may give a normal Y configuration of the commissures in diastole. Therefore it is not possible to exclude the diagnosis of bicuspid aortic valve just on diastolic images. In systole a normal valve will open to reveal a triangular shaped orifice as shown in Figure 5.4, whereas a functional or anatomically bicuspid valve will have an ellipsoid shaped orifice formed by the two leaflets (Figure 5.5). Therefore it is important to study the short axis leaflet configuration in both diastole and systole.

In late stage congenital aortic valve disease, calcification will occur on the valve leaflets. The intense echoes generated by the calcification will often obscure detail of valve leaflet anatomy. This can make it difficult to distinguish a bicuspid aortic valve from a rheumatic valve. However, at this stage of the disease process the exact etiology of the valve pathology is only of academic interest and will make little difference to the management of the case.

M-Mode echo is not as sensitive or specific as the 2D technique in diagnosing bicuspid aortic valves. The usual abnormality seen on the M-Mode is that the diastolic closure line

echo of the valve leaflets is eccentric. Therefore it is not placed centrally between the walls of the aortic root, as shown in Figure 5.6. Since 2D echo is so superior in establishing the diagnosis, M-Mode criteria in isolation should not be used.

Aortic stenosis results as the two commissures of the bicuspid valve progressively fuse and restrict the opening of the leaflets. Instead of opening wide and freely, the leaflets tend to dome (as with a stenotic mitral valve). This doming of the aortic valve can usually be seen in the long axis 2D image plane. An example is shown in Figure 5.7. Occasionally it is possible to appreciate doming in rheumatic aortic stenosis. However, when extensive calcification is present the exact configuration of the leaflets is again obscured.

Subaortic membrane is another form of congenital aortic stenosis. In this condition, a membrane partially covering the left ventricular outflow tract causes stenosis just below the aortic valve. The valve itself is usually normal. The membrane, which is very thin, can usually be visualized on 2D echo as shown in Figure 5.8. Sometimes it is easier to visualize the membrane using apical rather than parasternal views because the axial resolution of the imaging system will be higher than its lateral resolution. An example using apical views is seen in Figure 5.9.

In the young patient shown in Figure 5.8, the membrane is seen as a separate structure to the aortic valve. Left ventricular hypertrophy is also present. This suggests that the

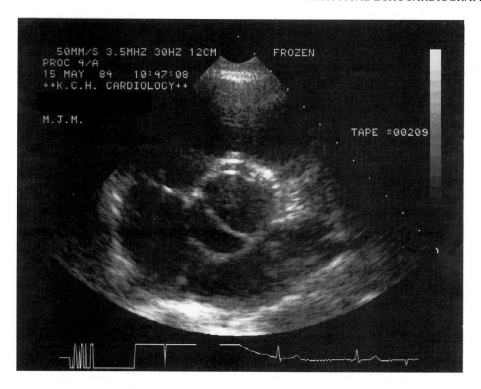

Figure 5.5 In this example of a bicuspid aortic valve the leaflets open during systole to reveal an ellipsoid shaped orifice.

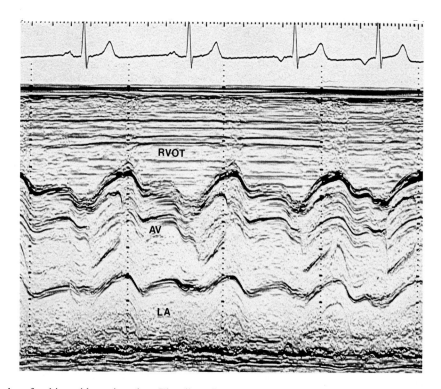

Figure 5.6 M-Mode echo of a bicuspid aortic valve. The diastolic closure line of the valve leaflets is eccentric and positioned more toward the anterior aortic root wall.

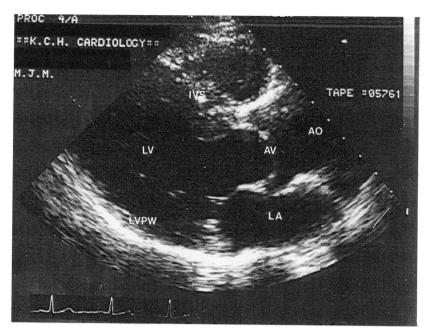

Figure 5.7 This long axis image shows systolic doming of the aortic valve leaflets in a young patient with a bicuspid valve. This type of doming is analogous to that seen in stenotic mitral valves where the leaflet edges are unable to separate completely.

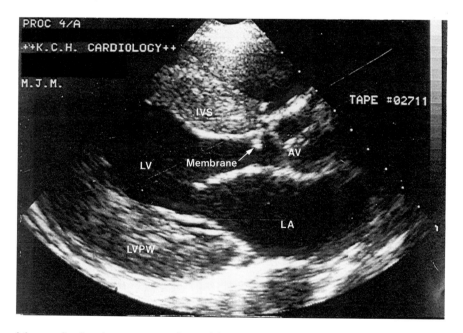

Figure 5.8 Parasternal long axis view in a young patient with a subaortic membrane. The membrane can be seen protruding into the left ventricular outflow tract from the interventricular septum, just beneath the aortic valve. There is considerable left ventricular hypertrophy, suggesting that the membrane may be highly stenotic.

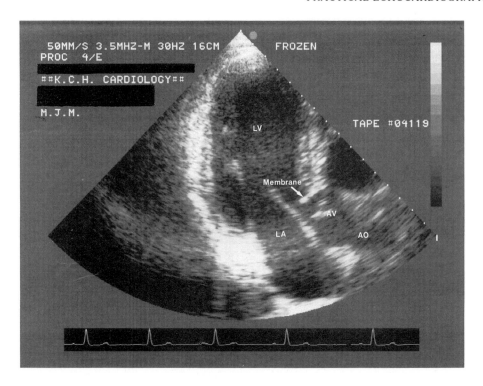

Figure 5.9 In this apical long axis view a subaortic membrane can be clearly visualized in the left ventricular outflow tract. It is separate from the aortic valve with a small subvalvar chamber between the membrane and the valve leaflets. In this view, the membrane is oriented perpendicular to the ultrasound pulses and is therefore more easily visualized than in parasternal views, where the orientation is parallel.

membrane is causing significant stenosis. Beyond the membrane the blood flow velocity will be high and turbulent. This results in marked systolic fluttering of the aortic valve as the turbulent blood passes through it. The fluttering can be seen on M-Mode echo and an example is shown in Figure 5.10. Echocardiography is one of the best available techniques for making this particular diagnosis, which can be very difficult on clinical criteria.

Congenital aortic valve disease is usually associated with aortic stenosis and/or incompetence. These hemodynamic conditions are obviously also present in acquired aortic valve disease and their assessment is discussed in the next section.

Acquired aortic valve disease

Aortic stenosis

As mentioned in Chapter 4, valvular calcification and fibrosis are easily detected by both M-Mode and 2D echoes. An aortic valve leaflet is usually considered abnormally thickened if it appears as thick as or thicker than the walls of the aortic root. The M-Mode appearance is that of mul-

tiple echoes occurring throughout the cardiac cycle due to calcification and corrugation on the valve leaflets and raphe.

Figure 2.8a demonstrates a normal aortic valve M-Mode recording. In contrast, Figures 5.11 and 5.12 illustrate increased valvular thickening due to fibrosis and calcification. In Figure 5.12 the calcification is so severe that the detail of the valve leaflets is completely obscured.

Increased aortic valve echoes secondary to aortic stenosis must be distinguished from other pathologies that can give similar appearances. Aortic atherosclerosis and vegetations due to endocarditis are examples. Careful and detailed examination technique will usually allow separation of the true valve leaflets from other structures which may give rise to misleading recordings. The echocardiographic appearances of aortic valve endocarditis are described in Chapter 9.

Using both M-Mode and 2D echoes in aortic stenosis it is also possible to appreciate the mobility and opening of the valve leaflets. With increasing valvular calcification the leaflets usually become less mobile. Unfortunately, the degree of calcification and the mobility/opening of the leaflets does not correlate reliably with the severity of aortic stenosis. However, if the aortic valve is heavily calcified and immobile, and left ventricular hypertrophy is seen, then it

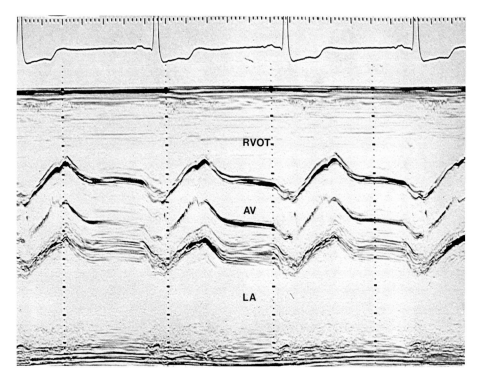

Figure 5.10 M-Mode echo of the aortic valve from the same patient illustrated in Figure 5.8. The aortic valve leaflets open at the beginning of systole and then almost completely close as turbulent high velocity blood flow caused by the membrane passes through them. This causes a fine systolic flutter of the valve leaflets which can be detected on M-Mode.

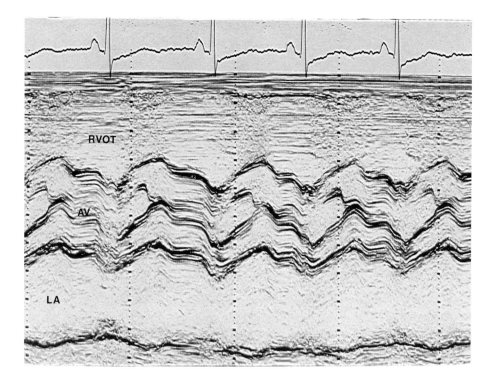

Figure 5.11 Aortic valve M-Mode echo in a patient with mild aortic stenosis. The valve leaflets exhibit some echo reduplication due to fibrosis and calcification; in addition, the separation of the leaflets in systole is reduced.

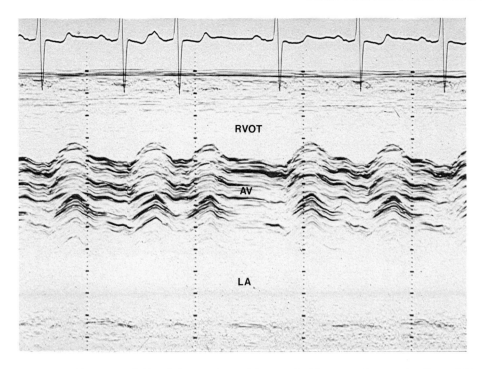

Figure 5.12 Severe valvular calcification and fibrosis in a patient with very significant aortic stenosis. The calcification is so extensive that the details of the valve anatomy and mobility are completely obscured.

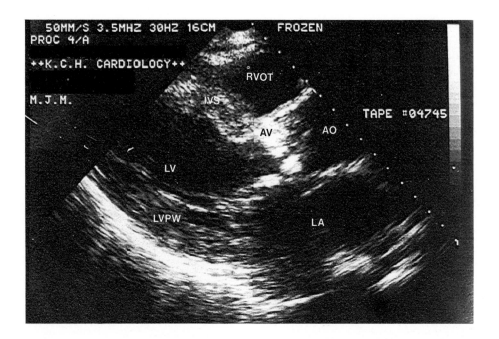

Figure 5.13 Parasternal long axis view in an elderly patient with severe calcific aortic stenosis. The calcified aortic valve leaflets are highly echo reflectant. The narrowed systolic orifice can be seen in this image. On real-time examination the leaflets appeared immobile and, in addition, there is left ventricular hypertrophy.

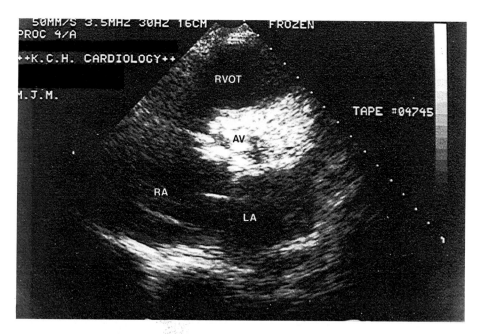

Figure 5.14 Short axis view of the aortic valve in the same patient illustrated in Figure 5.13. Again the valve leaflets appear very calcified and the leaflet anatomy is obscured.

is reasonable to assume that significant stenosis is present. Other causes of left ventricular hypertrophy such as hypertension must, of course, be excluded first.

On the M-Mode echo only the right coronary and noncoronary aortic valve leaflets are seen. This technique also obviously has a lack of spatial orientation which limits appreciation of the exact distribution of valvular calcification and mobility of the left coronary leaflet. These limitations are overcome to a large degree by the 2D technique. In Figures 5.13 and 5.14 the increased and thickened echoes from the calcified aortic leaflets can be seen. On the real-time moving 2D images the precise mobility of the leaflets could be appreciated. Left ventricular hypertrophy, secondary to the aortic stenosis, is also present in this example.

Attempts have been made to quantify the degree of aortic stenosis by directly measuring aortic valve area from the 2D echo. However, this has not proved successful because the orifice is usually so irregular and difficult to correctly identify. In addition, the clinical and hemodynamic gold standard for judging severity of stenosis is usually the transvalvar pressure gradient. Only a very small change in aortic valve area is required to produce a significant alteration in pressure gradient, and 2D echo does not have high enough resolution to quantify aortic valve area so precisely.

Doppler echocardiography (Chapter 11) facilitates measurement of aortic blood flow velocities. The velocity is increased in aortic stenosis and this can be used to accurately predict transvalvar pressure gradients and valve area.

Without Doppler, the severity of aortic stenosis cannot be reliably quantified by echo. However, it is possible to diagnose the condition and severe stenosis can usually be inferred by assessing the presence of left ventricular hypertrophy, the mobility of the valve leaflets and the extent of calcification and fibrosis.

Aortic incompetence

Aortic incompetence may occur in conjunction with aortic stenosis because the calcified and irregular valve leaflets are unable to coapt correctly in diastole. Incompetence is also found in endocarditis where the leaflets have become perforated (Figure 5.15) and in patients with dilatation of the valve annulus secondary to aortic root aneurysm or dissection, as shown in Figure 5.16.

Echocardiography plays a major role in determining the pathogenesis of the incompetence and also in monitoring left ventricular function. One of the primary effects of incompetence is to cause left ventricular volume overload. This manifests itself on the echo with the appearances of a dilated and hyperdynamic left ventricle. This can be

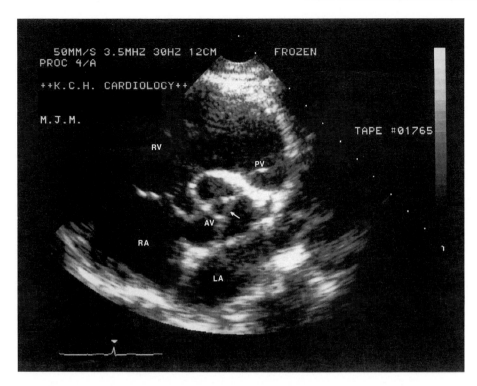

Figure 5.15   Short axis view of the aortic valve in a patient with severe aortic regurgitation secondary to aortic valve endocarditis. Perforation of the valve leaflets (arrowed) is seen in this image and a complete hole in the valve apparatus is evident.

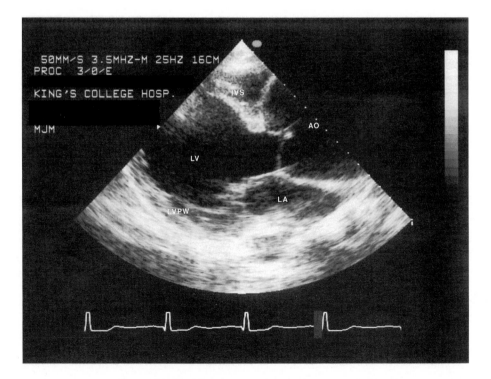

Figure 5.16a   Parasternal long axis view in a patient with an aortic root aneurysm. The aortic root is grossly dilated which, in turn, is causing stretching of the valve ring so that the leaflets no longer coapt completely in diastole, as seen in Figure 5.16b. The left ventricle is also dilated secondary to severe aortic regurgitation.

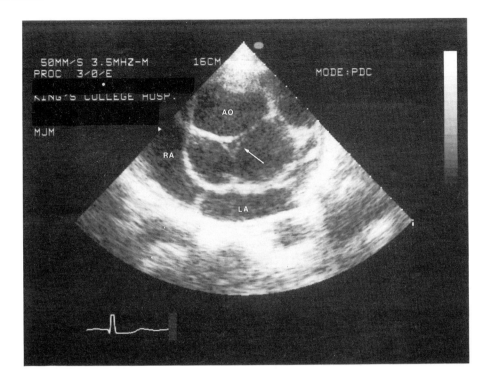

Figure 5.16b Short axis view of the aortic valve showing dilatation of the valve ring and inability of the leaflets to coapt in diastole, resulting in a regurgitant orifice (arrowed).

assessed with both 2D and M-Mode techniques. However, measurements of left ventricular size are more conveniently performed using the M-Mode, as described in Chapter 3.

Diagnosis of aortic incompetence is paradoxically performed by M-Mode examination of the mitral valve. The incompetent jet of blood very often strikes the mitral valve during diastole and causes one or both of the leaflets to flutter at high frequency. The flutter, which is superimposed upon the normal mitral valve motion, can be seen on the M-Mode recording, as in Figure 5.17. Occasionally the incompetent jet is directed toward the ventricular septum. In these cases it also possible to detect fine fluttering on the endocardial surface of the septum during diastole.

To the experienced observer, mitral valve flutter is a fairly specific indicator of aortic incompetence. However, the technique can lack sensitivity in patients with rheumatic mitral stenosis where the mitral valve leaflets are too rigid to flutter. If the incompetent jet is very eccentric, it may be directed away from both the mitral valve and septum and consequently be difficult to detect. Doppler echo has proved to be extremely sensitive and specific in the detection of aortic incompetence. It can also be used to quantify the degree of incompetence. This is not possible using conventional M-Mode or 2D echoes.

Many patients can tolerate even severe aortic incompetence for many years. However, they will deteriorate rapidly when left ventricular failure begins to occur. Echo provides

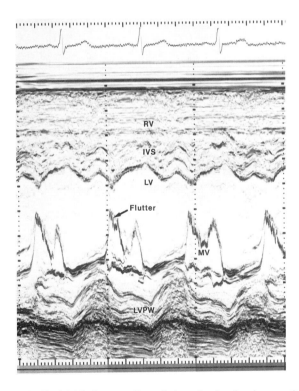

Figure 5.17 M-Mode recording of the mitral valve in a patient with aortic incompetence. Fine diastolic fluttering of the anterior mitral valve leaflet is seen. This is caused by the regurgitant jet from the aortic valve striking the mitral valve during diastole.

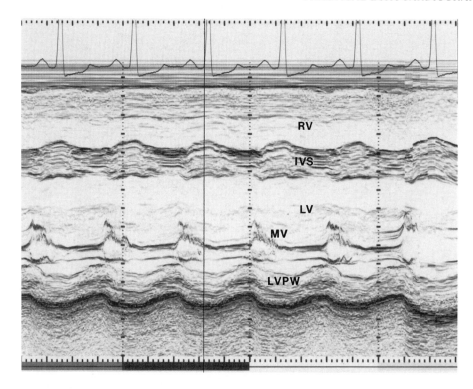

Figure 5.18 M-Mode recording of the left ventricle and mitral valve in a patient with severe, long-standing aortic incompetence. As shown, the mitral valve closes on the Q wave of the ECG and the left ventricle is dilated and contracting poorly. These findings are reputed to be poor prognostic indicators for aortic valve replacement.

a convenient method of following such patients serially. It is then possible to try to judge the best time to perform aortic valve replacement. Poor prognostic indicators include a left ventricular systolic dimension greater than 5.5 cm and/or early closure of the mitral valve (on or before the ECG R wave). Both these parameters are easily measured from the M-Mode echo and an example is shown in Figure 5.18.

Ideally, it is preferable to delay valve replacement as long as possible and yet still perform it while the prognosis is good. Regular echocardiographic monitoring of ventricular size, function and mitral valve closure should be carried out. Any sudden deterioration in these parameters, together with the clinical status, is currently the best indicator for timing of surgery.

Prosthetic aortic valves

The same general principles that were described in Chapter 4 for use in patients with mitral prostheses may be applied to prosthetic aortic valves.

Stenosis/obstruction of prosthetic valves is usually easier to appreciate in the tissue valves since it is normally possible to visualize the leaflets, which should appear thin and mobile. If they are thickened or calcified with a lack of

mobility, then stenosis of the valve must be considered. In prosthetic valves of the none tissue type, obstruction may be inferred if no or severely limited motion of the valve mechanism (ball or disc) is seen. especially if normal mobility has been previously documented on a baseline echo.

Both M-Mode and 2D echoes may be used to study the mobility of the valve leaflets and mechanism. However the 2D technique has obvious, previously described advantages. M-Mode echo can be used for timing the opening and closing of the valve, which may be useful in mild forms of obstruction where the only abnormality is delayed valve opening. Again, comparison with a baseline recording is very useful in detecting delayed opening.

Regurgitation of prosthetic aortic valves may be detected and evaluated in the same way as described for native valves. However, the regurgitant jets are often very eccentric and may not strike the mitral valve or septum, causing flutter, and prosthetic valve regurgitation can often be missed using conventional echocardiography. Doppler is a much more sensitive technique and is now considered mandatory in prosthetic valve evaluation. In patients with significant paravalvar leaks, excessive mobility of the valve sewing ring with respect to the aortic annulus may be seen. This obviously indicates partial dehiscence of the sewing ring and requires careful and detailed examination using 2D echo in multiple views.

CHAPTER 6

Cardiomyopathies

Echocardiography has greatly simplified the diagnosis and management of patients with cardiomyopathy. This chapter describes the echocardiographic findings in hypertrophic, restrictive and dilated (congestive) cardiomyopathies and explains the role that the technique now plays in the evaluation of these disorders.

Cardiomyopathies frequently masquerade as valvular, hypertensive, congenital or ischemic heart disease. The echocardiogram (both M-Mode and 2D echo) is a convenient noninvasive technique for making the true diagnosis

and very frequently suggesting the most suitable course of management.

Diffuse diseases of the heart muscle that do not have an etiology attributable to cardiac mechanical overload are classified as cardiomyopathies. Included in this classification are entities such as myocarditis (both viral and rheumatic) and myocardial depression secondary to toxic factors.

Cardiomyopathies can be categorized on the basis of anatomical and functional characteristics as illustrated in Figure 6.1. Dilated cardiomyopathies are characterized by

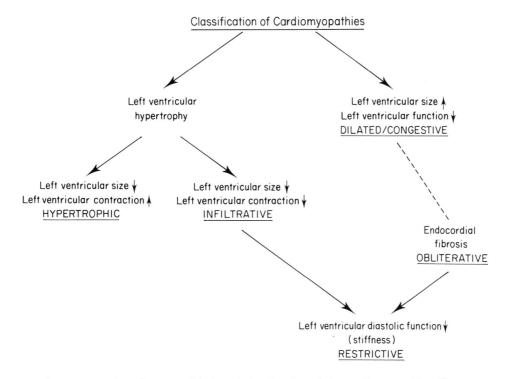

Figure 6.1 Diagrammatic representation of one possible broad classification of the cardiomyopathies. There are many variations and subdivisions of this classification not illustrated. For further description see the text.

dilatation and impairment of ventricular function. When hypertrophy of the ventricular walls is present the diagnosis of hypertrophic or infiltrative cardiomyopathy must be considered. In the latter case, ventricular function is usually reduced whereas in the hypertrophic cardiomyopathies the left ventricle is frequently hyperdynamic. Obliterative cardiomyopathies are associated with endocardial fibrosis and often partial obliteration of the left ventricular cavity. Both the obliterative and infiltrative forms of cardiomyopathy can result in myocardial stiffness and a reduction in left ventricular function; when this occurs the cardiomyopathies are considered to be restrictive.

The tremendous ability of echocardiography to demonstrate these functional and structural abnormalities has made the technique invaluable in diagnosing and differentiating between the different forms of cardiomyopathy.

Hypertrophic cardiomyopathy

Post-mortem studies indicate that the main diagnostic feature of hypertrophic cardiomyopathy is disproportionate thickening of the interventricular septum (asymmetric septal hypertrophy). Echocardiography is a unique means of demonstrating this in life.

Asymmetric septal hypertrophy is illustrated in Figure 6.2. This is an M-Mode echocardiogram of a patient with hypertrophic cardiomyopathy and the classical, very hypertrophied interventricular septum. In addition, the systolic thickening and motion of the septum is diminished, presumably as a result of the myocardial fiber disarray that is known to occur in this condition. The combination of septal hypertrophy, lack of motion and systolic thickening is one of the important echocardiographic indicators of hypertrophic cardiomyopathy. Although septal hypertrophy may occur in a variety of other conditions, such as hypertension, the septum is not usually also immobile.

The septal hypertrophy (in hypertrophic cardiomyopathy) is a primary cause of the reduced left ventricular cavity size also seen in Figure 6.2. Usually the septal hypertrophy tends to encroach upon the left ventricular outflow tract and this can be most easily evaluated using 2D echo.

The ratio of the septal thickness to that of the posterior left ventricular wall is an important diagnostic consideration. Henry et al. originally proposed that a ratio of greater than 1.3 : 1.0 should be considered diagnostic (the normal ratio is 1.03 : 1.0). However, a ratio of 1.5 : 1 is now generally used and this helps to minimize the number of false positives, although obviously reducing the sensitivity of this single criterion. In addition, the absolute thickness of the septum is of major importance and should be at least 1.4 cm

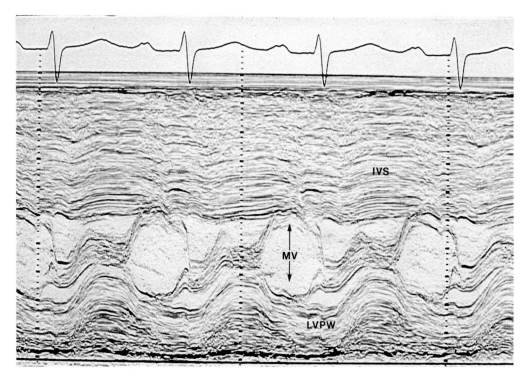

Figure 6.2 M-Mode recording from a patient with hypertrophic cardiomyopathy. The interventricular septum is grossly hypertrophied and it is difficult to distinguish its anterior surface. In addition the septum is immobile. The left ventricular cavity is small, particularly in systole.

in adults before a diagnosis of hypertrophic cardiomyopathy can be considered.

Trabeculation of the right side of the interventricular septum and/or echoes arising from the tricuspid valve apparatus can make identification of the true anterior septal surface difficult and lead to an overestimation of septal thickness. These problems can be overcome to a large degree by the use of 2D echo in combination with M-Mode. The spatial orientation afforded by the 2D technique greatly assists in identification of the true septal surface.

The use of 2D echo in this condition has confirmed previous post-mortem data that the distribution of septal and left ventricular hypertrophy in this condition may not be uniform. Indeed, it is now appreciated that patients with hypertrophic cardiomyopathy form a very heterogeneous population that can be subdivided into a number of different hypertrophic classifications dependent upon the distribution of hypertrophy. For example, the parasternal long axis view shown in Figure 6.3 demonstrates septal hypertrophy which extends to the region of the left ventricular outflow tract. In contrast, the subcostal four chamber view in Figure 6.4 illustrates apical septal hypertrophy which in systole causes left ventricular cavity obliteration at the apex. Therefore, in such cases of localized septal hypertrophy, the M-Mode measurement of septal thickness is obviously dependent upon exactly where the M-Mode beam traverses the septum. It is important to carefully examine the distribution of left ventricular hypertrophy in this condition (using all standard 2D views), since it can influence management and may possibly indicate surgical resection if outflow tract obstruction is caused by sub-aortic septal hypertrophy.

On the 2D echo the interventricular septum is usually strongly echo reflecting and has a "ground-glass" or "speckled" appearance. This again is almost certainly as a result of myocardial fiber disarray which provides many reflecting interfaces to the interrogating ultrasound beam, and is illustrated in Figures 6.5 and 6.6. In the latter example, the left ventricle has a banana-like shape; this is a common appearance. As on the M-Mode recording, the real-time 2D echo illustrates that the septum is usually immobile while the free walls of the ventricle have an exaggerated, hyperdynamic motion. The systolic cavity is very small and frequently completely obliterated. Sophisticated computer analysis of left ventricular contraction and relaxation patterns in this condition have shown that impairment of diastolic function is a common factor. Early research using computer analysis of echocardiograms has suggested that certain classes of drugs may reverse these diastolic abnormalities.

While asymmetric septal hypertrophy is almost always seen in hypertrophic cardiomyopathy, hemodynamic left ventricular outflow obstruction may or may not be present

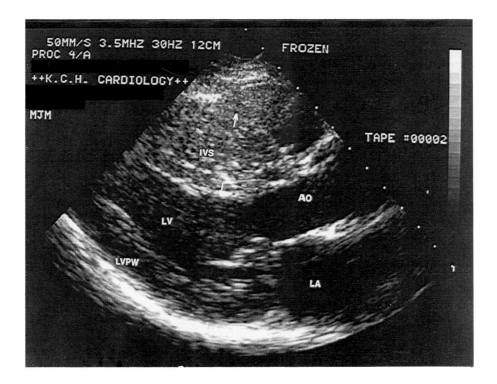

Figure 6.3 In this patient with hypertrophic cardiomyopathy, severe hypertrophy of the interventricular septum, extending from the left ventricular outflow tract toward the apex, is seen.

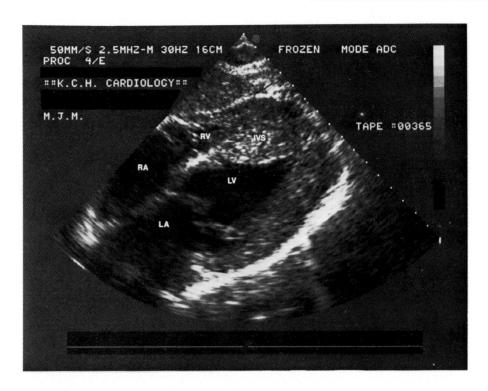

Figure 6.4   Subcostal four chamber view in a patient with "apical" hypertrophic cardiomyopathy. The apical regions of the right and left ventricle are very hypertrophied with some obliteration of the left ventricular cavity.

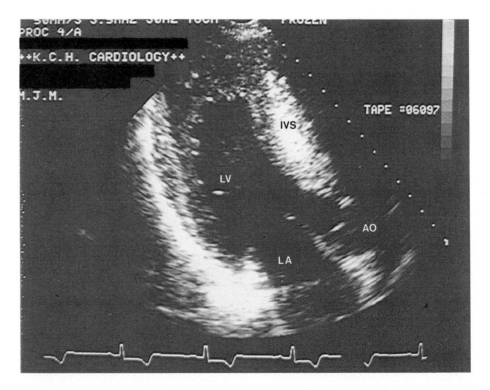

Figure 6.5   Apical long axis view in a patient with hypertrophic cardiomyopathy where myocardial fiber disarray has increased the reflectivity of the interventricular septum. This may occur to a lesser extent than illustrated here and the septum is described as having a "ground-glass" appearance.

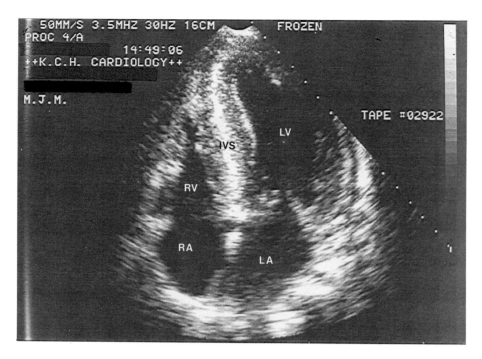

Figure 6.6 In this patient with hypertrophic cardiomyopathy the interventricular septum is, again, highly reflective. In addition, this apical four chamber view illustrates the "banana" shape of the left ventricle that is frequently described in this condition.

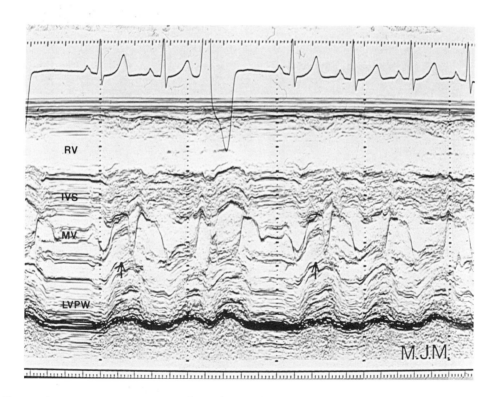

Figure 6.7 Systolic anterior motion of the mitral valve (arrowed) is seen on those sinus beats following the compensatory pause of ventricular ectopics. This illustrates the dynamic nature of this phenomenon and, in this case, is presumably due to postectopic accentuation of the intracavity gradient.

in this condition. One of the primary indicators of obstruction is systolic anterior motion of the mitral valve apparatus, as illustrated by the M-Mode recording in Figure 6.7. This abrupt displacement of the mitral valve leaflets toward the septum is probably the major cause of functional outflow obstruction. However, protrusion of the hypertrophied septum into the outflow tract is almost certainly another contributing factor. It has been suggested that the systolic anterior mitral valve movement may be caused by the hypertrophied papillary muscles extending into the left ventricular outflow tract when the ventricle shortens in systole, but it is also possible that the anterior cusp is sucked toward the septum as a result of the Venturi effect (Figure 6.8). Several studies using 2D echo have proposed both these conflicting theories as mechanisms for the systolic anterior mitral motion and this question has not been satisfactorily resolved. Since the left ventricular outflow obstruction is dynamic, it may not always be present at rest and therefore the systolic anterior motion will not be seen. In this group of patients it may only occur after a compensatory pause following a ventricular ectopic as shown in Figure 6.7. Alternatively it may be provoked by the Valsalva maneuver, amyl nitrate or isoprenaline.

Abnormal systolic motion of the aortic valve is also frequently seen in those patients with left ventricular outflow obstruction. As shown in Figure 6.9, this abnormal motion manifests itself as partial or complete midsystolic closure of the valve due to a sudden reduction and turbulence in ejection blood flow. While this finding enhances the reliability with which the diagnosis of obstruction may be made, it can also be seen in other conditions. Doppler examination of blood velocity in the outflow tract is very sensitive to both the presence and severity of hemodynamic obstruction. As Doppler equipment becomes widely available it will be undoubtedly accepted as a useful complementary technique in the assessment of hypertrophic cardiomyopathy.

None of the diagnostic features of hypertrophic cardiomyopathy described above are, in isolation, specific for this condition. However, when seen in combination the diagnosis must be strongly suspected.

Echocardiography plays a major role in studying the natural history of hypertrophic cardiomyopathy, in selecting patients who would be suitable for surgical resection of outflow obstruction and, as indicated previously, in evaluating the effects of drugs. Its noninvasive nature also makes it an ideal screening tool for examining the first-degree relatives of patients with this condition, which is genetically transmitted as a dominant trait. In these relatives only asymmetric septal hypertrophy is occasionally found, with none of the other classic hallmarks of hypertrophic cardiomyopathy. The significance of this finding is, as yet, unknown.

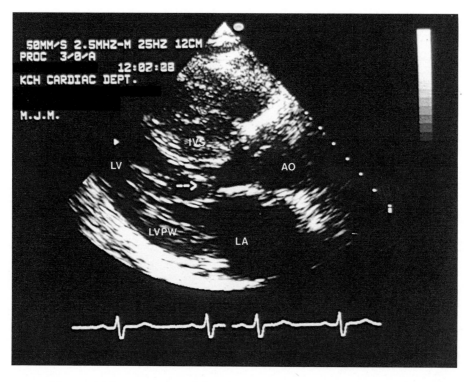

Figure 6.8 In this parasternal long axis view protrusion of the mitral valve apparatus and chordae (arrowed) into the left ventricular outflow tract during systole is seen. This is almost certainly the cause of the systolic anterior motion of the mitral valve seen on M-Mode recordings.

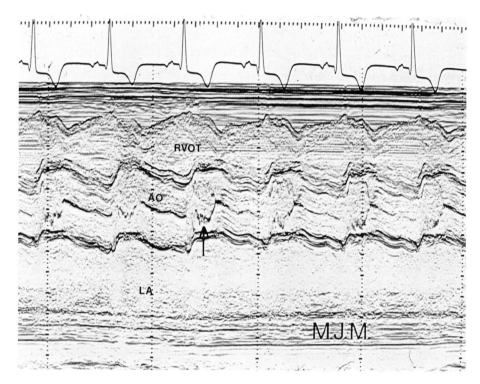

Figure 6.9 M-Mode recording of the aortic valve in a patient with hypertrophic obstructive cardiomyopathy. There is marked systolic fluttering and early closure (arrowed) of the aortic valve. This is due to turbulent and reduced blood flow secondary to obstruction in the left ventricular outflow tract.

Infiltrative cardiomyopathy

This relatively uncommon condition may arise secondary to disorders such as amyloidosis, collagen diseases, iron overload, sarcoidosis, glycogen storage disease and acromegaly, to name a few. The echo cardiac abnormalities found in these conditions usually present as marked cardiac hypertrophy and small ventricular cavities. In addition, ventricular wall motion is often decreased and a reduced mitral valve closure rate is evident on the M-Mode echocardiogram. This latter finding probably reflects a reduction in diastolic left ventricular compliance and ventricular filling rate as a result of the infiltration process. An M-Mode echocardiogram of a patient with amyloid infiltration of the heart is illustrated in Figure 6.10.

2D echocardiography has a useful role to play in the assessment of patients with this form of cardiomyopathy. It provides a more global appreciation of the extent of cardiac hypertrophy and ventricular wall motion. Hypertrophy of the interatrial septum, thickening of the atrioventricular valves and a patchy, heterogeneous distribution of echoes returning from the myocardium have been described using 2D echo in patients with amyloidosis. A 2D echo example of amyloid infiltrative cardiomyopathy is shown in Figure 6.11.

Echocardiographic evidence of both concentric and asymmetric left ventricular hypertrophy may be found in conditions other than hypertrophic and infiltrative cardiomyopathies. For example, left ventricular hypertrophy is well described in patients with hypertension or aortic stenosis and in athletes performing isometric exercise. These etiologies should be excluded before echocardiographic evidence of cardiac hypertrophy is attributed to cardiomyopathy.

Dilated (congestive) cardiomyopathies

Without echo the diagnosis of dilated cardiomyopathy can be difficult. For example, the chest X-ray of a patient with dilated cardiomyopathy may appear indistinguishable from the cardiomegaly seen in pericardial effusion. In addition, this form of cardiomyopathy may present with similar clinical findings to those of patients with hypertensive, valvar or ischemic heart disease. The differential diagnosis between dilated cardiomyopathy and these other disorders may usually be made with echocardiography.

However, the etiology of the cardiomyopathy cannot be determined from the echocardiogram. The technique can

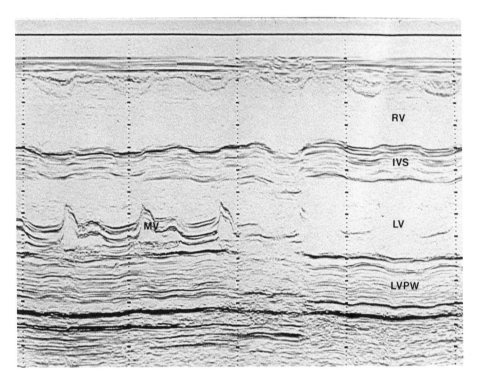

Figure 6.10 Some of the nonspecific features of amyloid infiltrative cardiomyopathy are illustrated in this M-Mode recording. The ventricular cavity is small with hypertrophied walls and, in addition, the wall motion is markedly reduced.

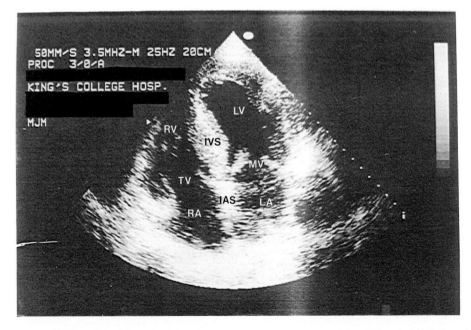

Figure 6.11 In this patient with amyloid infiltrative cardiomyopathy the interventricular septum is brightly echo reflectant, there is hypertrophy of the interatrial septum and the mitral valve appears thickened.

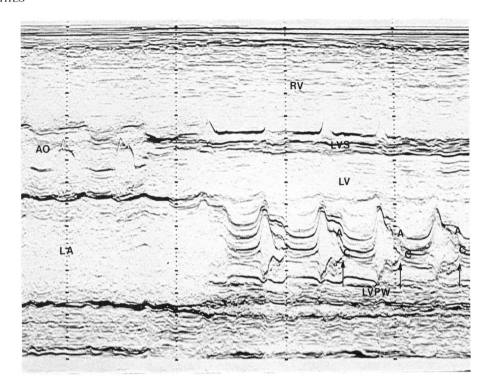

Figure 6.12 M-Mode scan from the aorta and left atrium through to the mitral valve. The left atrium, left ventricle and right ventricle are very dilated. The interventricular septum and posterior left ventricular wall contract very poorly and, in addition, there is delayed A–C closure of the mitral valve. This is indicative of a raised left ventricular end-diastolic pressure in this patient with dilated cardiomyopathy.

be very useful in assessing the degree of left ventricular dysfunction and for serial monitoring during treatment. For example, echocardiography can be easily used to document improvement in left ventricular function in patients with viral myocarditis following immunosuppressive therapy.

The M-Mode echocardiogram is usually sufficient for the diagnosis of dilated cardiomyopathy and will show a dilated, poorly contracting left ventricle. A typical M-Mode echo of a patient with dilated cardiomyopathy is seen in Figure 6.12.

On the echo the left ventricular diastolic internal dimension is normally greater than 5.6 cm in adults, this value being the accepted upper limit of normal. Septal and posterior left ventricular wall motion will be reduced and together these factors can be quantified by calculating the fractional shortening of the ventricle as described in Chapter 3.

Another useful M-Mode index of left ventricular function is to measure the separation between the mitral valve E point and the septum. This will normally be less than 1.5 cm and is inversely proportional to the ejection fraction. In a patient with dilated cardiomyopathy, the dilated left ventricle will increase the E point to septal separation. The low cardiac output will reduce the flow through the mitral valve and hence the extent of its opening, which will also increase the separation. These two factors combine to make the mitral E point to septal separation a very useful

index of left ventricular function, which can be conveniently used in a serial manner.

Delayed (A–C) closure of the mitral valve can also be seen on the M-Mode echo as seen in Figure 6.12. This is indicative of raised left ventricular end-diastolic pressure as a hemodynamic consequence of left ventricular failure. Other M-Mode features will frequently include a dilated right ventricle (when involved in the cardiomyopathy) and a dilated left atrium. The latter finding may be due directly to left ventricular failure and elevated ventricular filling pressure, or to functional mitral regurgitation caused by dilatation of the mitral valve annulus. When mitral regurgitation is present it can be difficult to determine if it has occurred secondary to left ventricular dilatation (as in congestive cardiomyopathies) or whether it is itself the primary factor and the dilated left ventricle has resulted from volume overload. In the latter case the mitral valve may appear abnormal, and the left ventricular function will be better than in patients with dilated cardiomyopathy.

Septal and posterior left ventricular wall thickness is usually normal, although myocardial mass is increased due to dilatation. Fibrous replacement of the diseased myocardium may occur and this will lead to very dense echoes which can often be seen on both the M-Mode and 2D echoes.

The 2D echo, as shown in Figure 6.13, will also demonstrate the dilated, poorly contracting left and perhaps right ventricle. The 2D technique does allow a better, overall appreciation of wall motion than M-Mode and hence is superior for detecting segmental dysfunction; again multiple views should be utilized. Segmental dysfunction can occur, for example, in patients with focal viral myocarditis where at some stages of the pathology only part of the ventricular wall may be involved.

As described in Chapter 3, it is possible to calculate the ejection fraction from the 2D echo and use it to document left ventricular function. This technique is more applicable when segmental dysfunction is present because the M-Mode alone can be misleading in these cases.

Mural thrombi are relatively common in dilated cardiomyopathies, especially in those of viral origin (Figure 6.14).

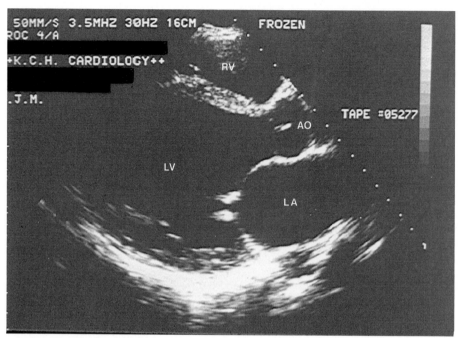

Figure 6.13 Parasternal long axis view in a young patient with dilated cardiomyopathy secondary to acute viral myocarditis. There is significant dilatation of the left ventricular cavity and also the left atrium. In addition, on the moving real-time images, diffuse hypokinesis of the ventricular walls could be seen on all 2D image planes.

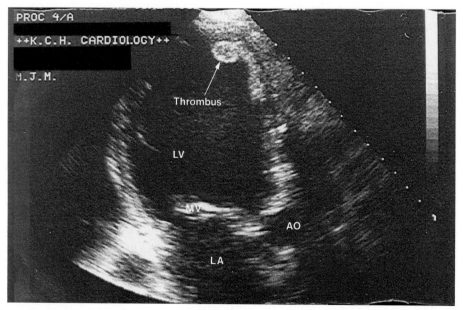

Figure 6.14 Apical long axis view in another patient with viral myocarditis. In the anteroapical region of the left ventricle a brightly echo reflectant pedunculated thrombus is seen. The spherical tip of the thrombus was highly mobile and considered to be at risk for embolization.

As described in Chapter 9, the 2D echo is quite a sensitive technique for detecting thrombus. When thrombus is seen it is usually considered to be an indication for anticoagulation. However, trabeculation of the left ventricle can occur in this form of cardiomyopathy and may be confused with mural thrombus. This factor must be considered before a diagnosis of thrombus (in patients with dilated cardiomyopathy) can be made.

The etiology of dilated cardiomyopathy may range from viral myocarditis, alcohol abuse, postpartum or idiopathic origins. To date, echocardiography has not been successful in predicting the individual cause but has been very useful in establishing the diagnosis and in following the efficacy of therapy or the natural history of the condition.

CHAPTER 7

Coronary artery disease

The tremendous ability of echocardiography to visualize the structure and function of the ventricular cavities has made this technique a very useful tool to study the effects of myocardial ischemia and infarction resulting from coronary artery disease.

It has been appreciated for some time that using high quality 2D echocardiographic equipment it is possible to image the origins of both the left and right coronary arteries. An example showing the left main coronary artery is seen in Figure 7.1. Several case reports have described the detection of proximal coronary artery lesions using 2D echo, although the specificity of the technique in this role is currently too low to be of routine clinical use.

In addition, it is possible to measure blood flow rates in the left coronary artery using combined Doppler and echo techniques and these measurements have been correlated with invasive assessments of coronary status. Again, these are still experimental applications of echocardiography, but it is likely that in the future they will find a useful role.

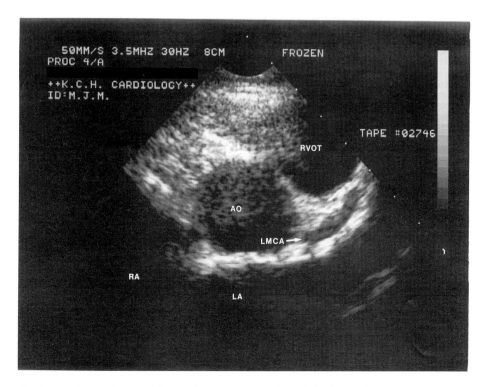

Figure 7.1 Short axis view of the aortic root showing the proximal portion of the left main coronary artery arising from the aorta.

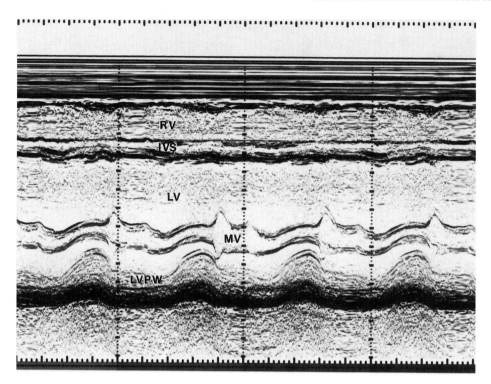

Figure 7.2   M-Mode echo of the left ventricle in a patient with anteroseptal myocardial infarction. The interventricular septum is akinetic (not contracting), whereas the posterior left ventricular wall exhibits normal motion. In addition, the left ventricular cavity is dilated.

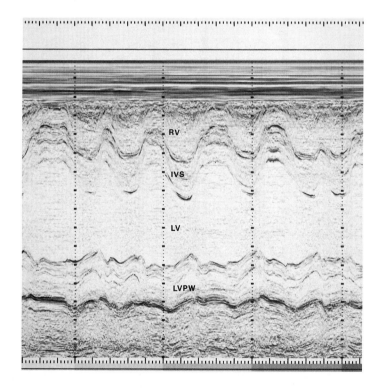

Figure 7.3   In this M-Mode echo, the posterior left ventricular wall is hypokinetic (moving poorly), which is consistent with a posterior myocardial infarct. The interventricular septum is hyperkinetic (exaggerated motion) which is a compensatory phenomenon frequently seen in noninfarct segments.

Acute myocardial infarction and ischemia

One of the earliest consequences of myocardial ischemia is abnormal contraction and systolic thickening of the ischemic area. In experimental studies, this has been shown to occur within 10 beats of the onset of ischemia, long before electrocardiographic or cardiac enzyme abnormalities. Since echocardiography is an ideal technique for studying wall motion and thickening it can be very useful in documenting the presence and extent of ischemia and infarction, even in the very early stages. This is of great relevance if therapy to limit the size of an infarct is being considered, since the success of this type of treatment is dependent on its early institution.

The M-Mode echo is clearly limited to evaluation of the septum and posterior left ventricular walls. As previously mentioned, the results of ischemia and/or infarction in these areas can be seen as a lack of systolic thickening and

contraction of the involved region. Figures 7.2 and 7.3 illustrate cases of anteroseptal and posterior myocardial infarction respectively. Where abnormal septal motion (from ischemia) is seen, as in Figure 7.2, this is usually indicative of significant obstruction in the left main or proximal left anterior descending coronary artery. Unfortunately, it has not been possible to correlate other areas of wall motion abnormalities with the site of coronary artery lesions in the same way, presumably due to the normal variability of coronary anatomy and the presence of any collateral circulation.

The 2D echo affords a more complete and spatially oriented view of left ventricular function than M-Mode. It is therefore more applicable in the evaluation of ischemia and infarction. A suggested nomenclature for the identification of myocardial wall segments using 2D views is shown in Figure 7.4. On the real-time, moving 2D image it is usually fairly easy to appreciate areas of myocardium that are failing to contract and move in systole. These areas can be related to the suggested nomenclature.

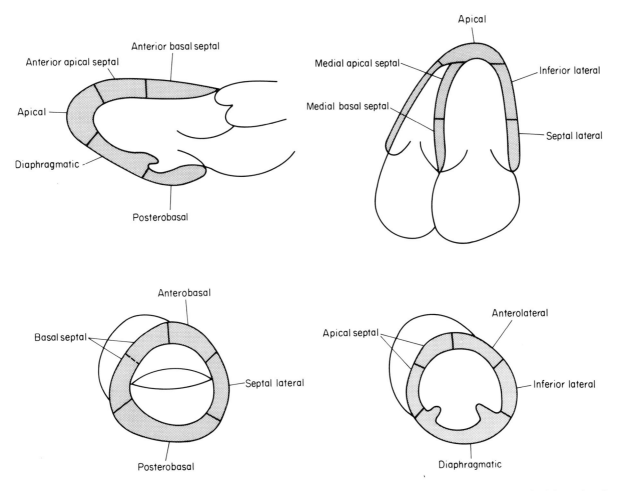

Figure 7.4 A suggested nomenclature for identification of myocardial wall segments. Parasternal long axis, apical four chamber, and two parasternal short axis planes are illustrated. Some segments will obviously be common to several image planes.

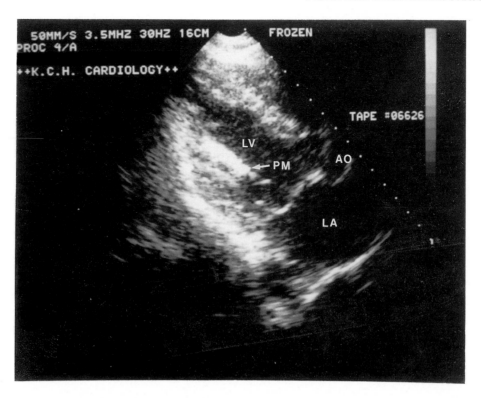

Figure 7.5   Long axis view of the left ventricle with the transducer positioned midway between the left sternal edge and the cardiac apex. In this patient, who has had an extensive inferior infarct, the papillary muscles are scarred and highly echo reflectant because of fibrous tissue. This patient also had mitral regurgitation as a result of the papillary muscle dysfunction.

Wall motion abnormalities may be categorized in different ways. The most popular and familiar method is to describe segments as either hypokinetic (moving poorly), akinetic (not moving) or dyskinetic (moving outwards in systole). Wall motion abnormalities can occur in patients with conduction abnormalities (especially if being paced) and also when the whole heart is moving in patients with large pericardial effusions. In addition, an obvious tethering effect exists between adjacent myocardial segments, so that wall motion in one segment is influenced by motion (or lack of it) in adjoining segments. For these reasons, lack of systolic thickening and even systolic thinning of myocardial segments is considered to be a more sensitive and specific indicator of ischemia/infarction. Good quality, high resolution 2D images with good endocardial definition are clearly needed in order to reliably document wall motion and thickening.

The total extent of echo documented wall motion abnormalities in patients with acute myocardial infarction does correlate well with final prognosis. Several centers now use the technique in their coronary care units as part of the routine evaluation of patients admitted with suspected or confirmed infarction, the obvious advantage being the ability to perform serial noninvasive examinations which can evaluate expansion of ischemia and infarction, and also the effect of drugs.

Scar tissue from old myocardial infarction is usually a very strong reflector of ultrasound due to its high collagen content. It is therefore frequently possible to localize areas of myocardial scarring, as shown in Figure 7.5. In this particular case the papillary muscles were scarred and caused significant mitral valve regurgitation.

While scar tissue is relatively easy to detect on the standard echocardiogram, several experimental studies have indicated that more subtle modifications to the reflected ultrasound may occur in areas of acutely ischemic myocardium. These effects are too small to be seen in a standard image but can be quantified by sophisticated computer analysis of the returning ultrasound. This technique is known as tissue characterization and may eventually provide us with a whole new dimension in echocardiography where areas of abnormal and ischemic heart muscle will be displayed upon a coloured image in a different hue to that of normal myocardium.

Myocardial contrast echocardiography has been recently used to demonstrate perfusion defects within the myocardium. This technique utilizes specially prepared echo-reflectant contrast medium (containing microspheres) that may be injected directly into the coronary arteries, the aorta, or even intravenously, to opacify the myocardium and reveal areas of abnormal perfusion. This new technique clearly has tremendous potential for the future.

Complications of myocardial infarction

The major role currently played by echocardiography in coronary artery disease is in the evaluation of complications of myocardial infarction. These complications may range from pericardial effusion associated with Dressler's syndrome to acute rupture of the mitral valve chordae and papillary muscles, resulting in severe mitral regurgitation.

In the latter case, the differential diagnosis between postinfarct acute mitral regurgitation and ventricular septal defect can obviously be difficult on both clinical and auscultatory examination. The 2D echo is usually able to provide a convenient and immediate method of diagnosis and will also allow appreciation of residual left ventricular function.

Acute mitral regurgitation will be evident by a bizzare motion of the mitral valve leaflets which, with the ruptured chordae, may prolapse back into the left atrium in systole. In addition, there will usually be dilatation of the left atrium, which is accommodating the regurgitant blood, and also a hyperdynamic left ventricle compensating for the regurgitation (as described in Chapter 4). Using Doppler techniques it is also possible to detect and quantify the regurgitant jet within the left atrium, as described in Chapter 11.

Postinfarct ventricular septal defects can often be directly visualized on the 2D echo image; a clear hole or discontinuity in the septum may be seen. Examples are illustrated in Plate 7.1 and Figures 7.6a and b. In both these cases, the echo has made the diagnosis, sited the defect and confirmed that left ventricular function is good. This provided enough information for surgery to proceed without further investigation, as is frequently the case. It is usually possible to reliably site the defect and this will influence the timing of surgery. The position of the defect will also affect the kind of surgical approach undertaken. Unfortunately, some postinfarct septal defects do not have a clear, discrete hole which is easy to visualize. In these cases it can be difficult to make the diagnosis from conventional echo without the assistance of Doppler, particularly color flow mapping.

Another complication of myocardial infarction is that of left ventricular aneurysm, and a technically satisfactory 2D echo is probably the definitive examination for excluding or detecting this condition. There are no consistent charac-

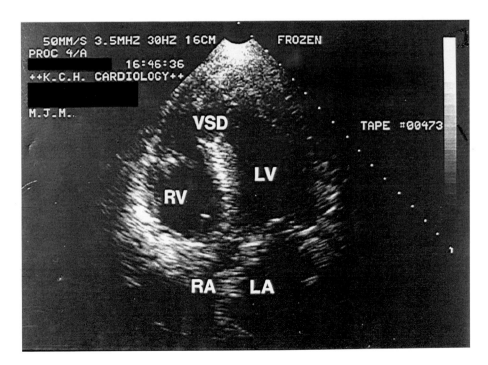

Figure 7.6a   Apical four chamber view of the patient in Plate 7.1. A large postinfarct ventricular septal defect is seen in the interventricular septum near the cardiac apex.

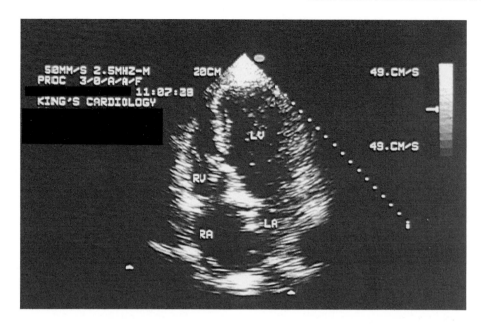

Figure 7.6b   A postinfarct ventricular septal defect in the mid portion of the interventricular septum is seen in this apical four chamber view. The septum exhibits a 1 cm discontinuity with displacement of part of the septal structure into the right ventricle.

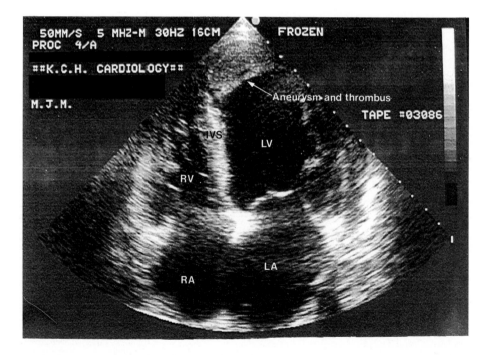

Figure 7.7   Apical four chamber view in a patient with an apical left ventricular aneurysm which has become almost totally filled with laminated thrombus.

teristic ECG, X-ray or physical findings that confirm the diagnosis. Frequently patients with an aneurysm are difficult to manage and have a mortality of about 60% over three years. Since this lesion is frequently amenable to surgery, the echocardiogram has become very important in establishing a noninvasive diagnosis, which can lead to left ventricular angiography in selected cases.

The typical appearance of left ventricular aneurysm may be seen in Figures 7.7 and 7.8. The normal diastolic contour of the left ventricular cavity has been interrupted by a bulging area of infarcted muscle that is frequently dyskinetic with the aneurysmal area moving outwards in systole instead of contracting inwards. Blood stasis commonly occurs within the aneurysm and this predisposes to thrombus formation. Fortunately this can usually be visualized on the echo examination and may warrant anticoagulation (see Chapter 9).

In addition to establishing the diagnosis of an aneurysm, the echo can also be used to determine whether the aneurysm is discrete or involves a large portion of the left ventricle. How much of the myocardium still contracts well and remains viable is obviously prognostically important and, together with the size and location of the aneurysm, is an indicator of the suitability for surgery.

Aneurysms are most commonly sited at the left ventricular apex but may occur in other positions. Pseudo-aneurysms are bordered by pericardium rather than by scarred and infarcted myocardium. Since they occur through rupture of the free ventricular wall, they usually have a narrow neck and the aneurysm can be seen extending behind the wall as shown in Figure 7.9.

The useful role that echocardiography can play in the management of patients with coronary artery disease is underestimated in many centers. As the applications of the technique in this condition become more widely appreciated, echocardiographic equipment will become a more common sight in coronary care units and it may eventually be deemed a mandatory investigation for all patients with suspected or confirmed ischemic heart disease.

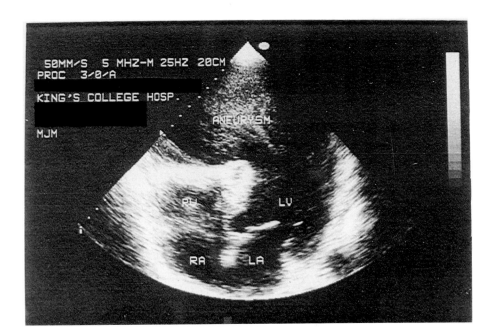

Figure 7.8 A very large apical and anterior left ventricular aneurysm is seen in this patient in whom the remaining left ventricular function was well preserved. Spontaneous "cloud-like" echoes are seen within the aneurysm as a result of blood stasis and red blood cell aggregation.

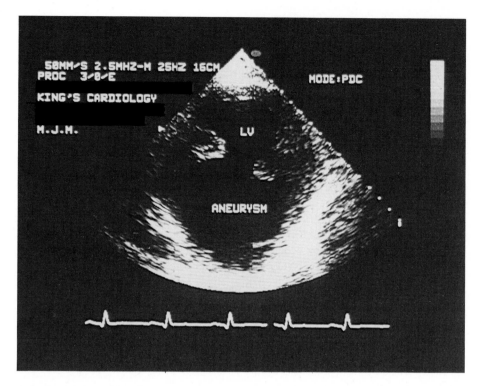

Figure 7.9 Parasternal short axis view of the left ventricle demonstrating a large pseudo-aneurysm behind the posterior/inferior wall. Although the aneurysm is large, it has a narrow neck connecting it to the true left ventricular cavity, and this helps to confirm that it is indeed a pseudo- rather than a true aneurysm.

CHAPTER 8

Pericardial effusion

Echocardiography is undoubtedly the technique of choice for the diagnosis of pericardial effusions. It has a very high sensitivity and accuracy. In addition, it may be used at the bedside, unlike other techniques.

Normally, the heart is in direct contact with the pericardial sac with no more than 10–20 ml of fluid in the potential cavity between the two structures. Fluid forming a pericardial effusion can accumulate in the pericardial cavity for a wide variety of reasons. If the quantity of fluid is small or it collects slowly, the pericardium is usually able to stretch to accommodate the extra volume. However, if the pericardium is noncompliant or a larger quantity of fluid accumulates acutely, for example in myocardial hemorrhage or rupture, then the function of the heart will be severely compromised by the external pressure exerted upon it. Cardiac tamponade will then result and prompt aspiration of the fluid is usually required.

Tamponade can sometimes be recognized on the echocardiogram as a diastolic collapse of the right ventricle. This occurs when the intrapericardial pressure exceeds the pressure within the right heart (in diastole) and causes the right ventricle to collapse. This is easiest to appreciate using real-time 2D images. Diastolic right atrial collapse has also been proposed as an indicator of cardiac tamponade. However, this finding is almost certainly over-sensitive and lacks specificity. Unfortunately, right ventricular collapse, while being more specific, is not a very sensitive indicator of tamponade.

As previously discussed, on both M-Mode and parasternal 2D echo the pericardium is usually seen as a very dense echo behind the posterior left ventricular wall. An example of a normal M-Mode echo is shown in Figure 8.1. When pericardial fluid is present it generates an echo free space between the pericardium and the heart. The fluid tends to gravitate posteriorly and therefore small to moderate effusions are usually most easily seen behind the posterior left ventricular wall, as in Figure 8.2.

It is unusual for pericardial fluid to collect behind the left atrium because the pericardium is reflected away from the left atrial wall by the pulmonary veins. Indeed, one of the distinguishing features between pleural and pericardial effusions is that in the latter case a posterior echo free space is unlikely to extend behind the left atrium. In a pleural effusion, fluid is often seen behind the left atrium. On 2D long axis views it is possible to visualize the descending aorta posterior to the pericardium, as in Figure 8.3. If the echo free space from an effusion is seen anterior to the aorta then it is almost certainly a pericardial rather than pleural effusion (Figures 8.4 and 8.5).

Small pericardial effusions are often only seen using 2D echo. With larger effusions, fluid will collect all around the heart and on the M-Mode an echo free space will be seen anteriorly as well as posteriorly. Occasionally the volume of fluid will be large enough to allow the heart to swing within the pericardial cavity. This swinging motion can be seen on the M-Mode in Figure 8.6. It can result in electrical alternans on the ECG recording as the heart continuously changes its position within the body. The swinging movement of the heart is superimposed upon normal cardiac motion and this makes it impossible to comment upon cardiac function while such a large effusion remains.

M-Mode echocardiography is limited to assessment of anterior or posterior collections of pericardial fluid. However, 2D obviously affords a more complete evaluation of the extent and distribution of fluid and this is particularly pertinent if the effusion is loculated. Multiple 2D echo views are used to examine the potential pericardial cavity and localize echo free spaces that would indicate the presence of fluid. Fibrinous membranes that would form loculations can be directly visualized on the 2D image. Their presence makes pericardiocentesis difficult, since all the loculations have to be entered by the drainage catheter to effect complete evacuation of fluid. In Figure 8.7 a short axis 2D image of a patient with a moderate size effusion is

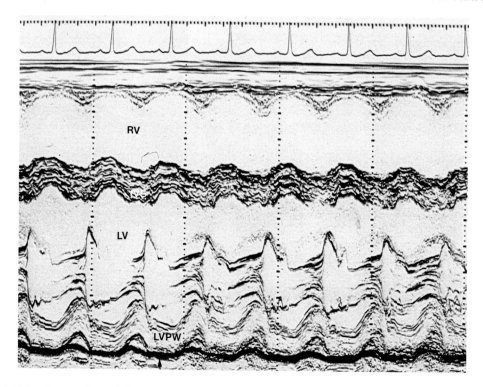

Figure 8.1 Normal M-Mode recording of the left ventricle. The dense, dark echo from the pericardium is seen posteriorly. In systole a small separation occurs between the pericardium and the epicardial surface of the posterior left ventricular wall. This is a normal finding and represents the small quantity of pericardial fluid that normally exists. In addition, the pericardium normally moves slightly anteriorly in systole as shown in this example.

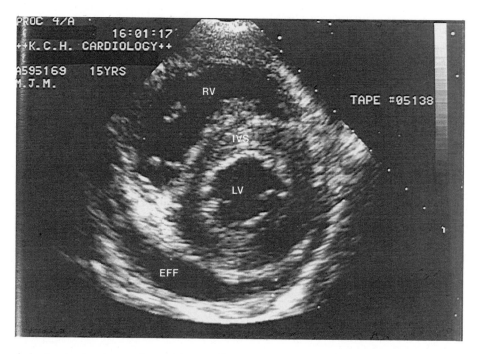

Figure 8.2 Parasternal short axis view in a patient with a small pericardial effusion. Small effusions tend to gravitate posteriorly, as demonstrated in this example.

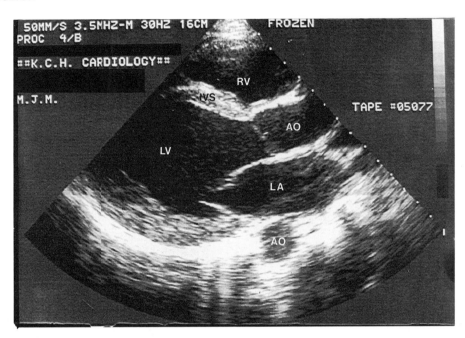

Figure 8.3 Parasternal long axis view in a normal patient. The very bright posterior echo generated by the pericardium runs anterior to the descending aorta, which is situated posterior to the left atrium.

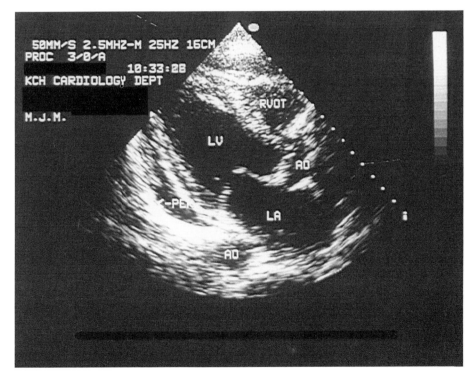

Figure 8.4 In this long axis view of the heart an echo free space is seen behind the posterior left ventricular wall. This is identified as a pericardial effusion since the pericardium can be seen situated anterior to the descending aorta.

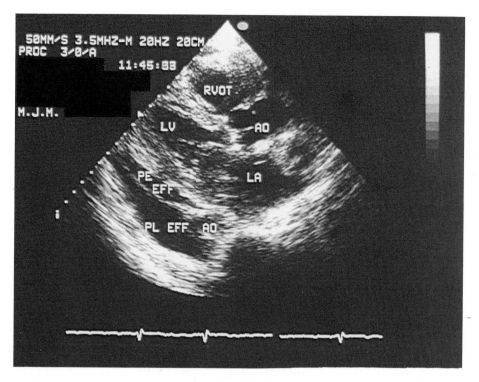

Figure 8.5 In this patient, pericardial and pleural effusions can be seen behind the heart. Again it is possible to identify the position of the pericardium by examining the orientation of the descending aorta with respect to the echo free spaces.

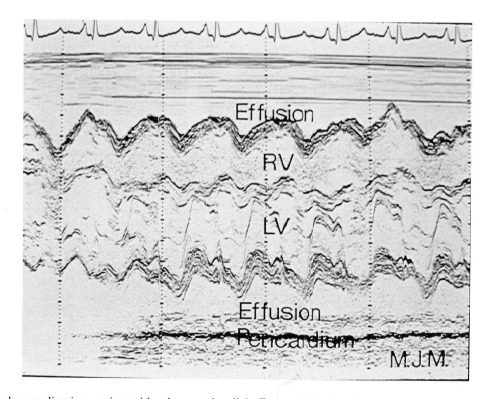

Figure 8.6 M-Mode recording in a patient with a large pericardial effusion. Echo free spaces are seen both anterior and posterior to the heart. In addition, a swinging motion of the heart can be seen as it moves anteriorly and posteriorly within the pericardial cavity. This motion can distort intracavity structures and in this patient artefactually suggests late systolic mitral valve prolapse.

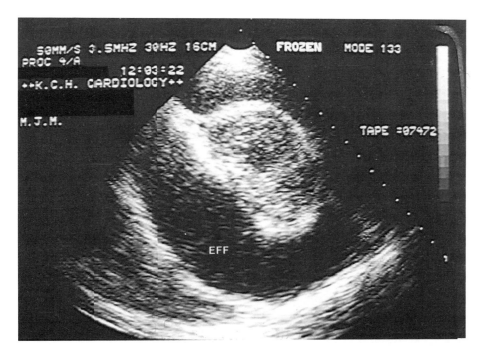

Figure 8.7 Short axis view of a large loculated pericardial effusion. A fibrous band attaches the anteromedial aspect of the heart to the pericardium. A large echo free space is seen surrounding the remainder of the heart.

seen. On the anteromedial aspect of this image a fibrinous band or membrane connecting the heart and pericardium is visualized. However, this was the only membrane visualized in all the 2D echo views and it did not hamper the aspiration of fluid. In Figure 8.8 multiple membranes in the pericardial cavity can be seen. This indicates extensive loculation and therefore drainage by traditional pericardiocentesis would be very difficult. Occasionally structures within the pericardial cavity will appear not as membranes but as distinct masses, often moving randomly within the fluid. The etiology and significance of these masses is uncertain; however, they are probably thrombi and/or fibrinous plaques.

Using 2D echo images it is possible to semiquantitate the amount of pericardial fluid present, provided it is not loculated. Quantification is usually performed with the parasternal long axis and/or apical four chamber views. Most types of 2D echo equipment have a facility which allows the user to measure the volume of a given portion of the image. It is possible to trace into the machine, from the 2D image, the approximate outer border of the heart and separately the pericardial margin which contains both fluid and the heart. If the heart volume, calculated by the equipment, is then subtracted from the total pericardial volume, the remaining figure is an approximation to the quantity of fluid present. An example utilizing a four chamber view is shown in Figure 8.9. Ideally, the mean volume calculated from both the four chamber and long axis views should be used.

In practice, this technique usually provides a volume that is accurate to within 50–100 ml. This estimate is certainly superior to guesswork and it does provide an indication of the amount of fluid that can be expected to be aspirated.

If the 2D echo examination is performed with the patient in the same position as they would be for a pericardiocentesis procedure, it is possible to choose the best site for insertion of the aspiration needle. This is usually performed subcostally or from the apex. With the echo transducer placed in both positions, the site with maximum separation between pericardial and cardiac epicardial surfaces is chosen. A distance of at least 1 cm is essential to reduce the risk of the aspiration needle puncturing the myocardium. In Figure 8.9 there is only a short distance between the pericardium and the myocardium over the cardiac apex, whereas in the subcostal view shown in Figure 8.10 there is a much larger and safer separation. When the least hazardous position has been selected, it is usually possible to position the transducer within a few centimetres of the needle and directly visualize its progress through the chest wall into the pericardial cavity. Although this technique requires the use of a sterilized transducer and sterile ultrasound coupling gel, it does make pericardiocentesis less hazardous and allows continuous monitoring of the remaining pericardial fluid.

Although the detection of pericardial effusions by echocardiography is comparatively easy, the technique has not met with the same degree of success in the assessment

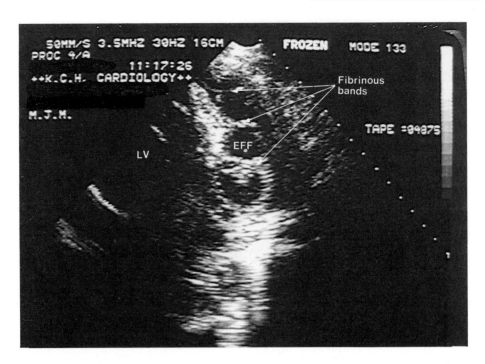

Figure 8.8   Short axis view demonstrating the fibrous bands within the pericardial cavity in a patient with multiple pericardial loculations.

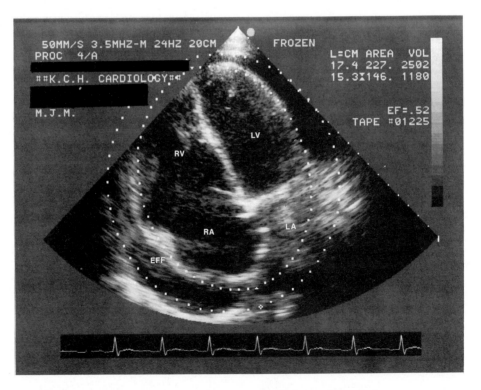

Figure 8.9   A typical four chamber view in a patient with a large pericardial effusion. The effusion appears to surround most of the heart and its volume is estimated by using the volume calculation package within the echo equipment. The volume of the entire pericardial cavity enclosing the heart is calculated to be 2500 ml and the volume of the heart itself is 1180 ml. By subtracting one from the other, the volume of the effusion is approximately 1300 ml. This procedure should be repeated using long axis views and an average of the two figures taken.

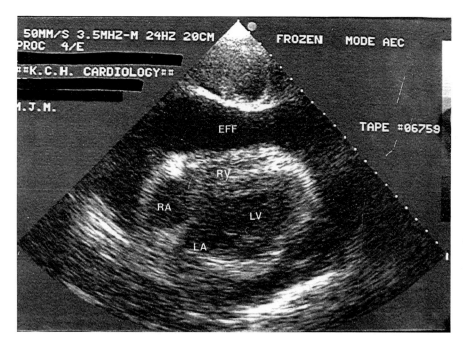

Figure 8.10 In this subcostal view there is a separation of approximately 3 cm between the pericardium and the epicardial surface of the right ventricular free wall. This gap should provide a large safety margin for a subcostal approach for the fluid aspiration.

of other pericardial lesions. While it is usually possible to comment upon the presence of pericardial thickening, constrictive pericarditis can be difficult to evaluate. Alterations in right ventricular size with respiration may be seen in constrictive pericarditis, but this finding is not very sensitive or specific.

Absence of respiratory variation in vena cava diameter is another indicator of constriction that appears to be useful. If the inferior vena cava is visualized using subcostal views it will be noted that its diameter decreases during inspiration in normal patients. Where constriction is present there appears to be no reduction in vessel diameter during inspiration.

Current research using Doppler echocardiography to study ventricular filling patterns in constriction appears very hopeful. This may extend the current role of echo to the evaluation of the complete spectrum of pericardial disorders.

CHAPTER 9

Intracardiac masses

The most dramatic echocardiographic images are often provided by visualization of masses within the heart. This chapter demonstrates examples of such structures and explains how echocardiography can be used in the diagnosis and management of patients who have differing types of intracardiac masses.

Thrombi, cardiac tumors and vegetations secondary to infective endocarditis are the three major causes of intracardiac masses. Once greater than 2–3 mm in size, these masses are usually detectable by echocardiography providing their density differs from the surrounding medium (usually blood). Obviously, the image quality and resolution of the echo equipment will affect its ability to image small homogeneous masses.

Infective endocarditis

Valvular vegetations arising from endocarditis are best detected and evaluated by 2D echo rather than M-Mode. The incidence of echo visible vegetations in proven endocarditis is about 50%. Therefore, the technique is not cost-effective when being used as a tool to establish a diagnosis of endocarditis. However, when vegetations can be seen, it does have an important role to play.

Vegetations less than 2–3 mm in size are below the resolving limit of most equipment. In addition, certain valves are difficult to visualize and the pre-existence of valvar disease may make the diagnosis difficult. However, the presence of echo detectable vegetations is of clinical importance because it does signify significant valve tissue destruction. Several studies have demonstrated that the size of vegetations is roughly proportional to the incidence of multiple embolic events. In addition, it is unusual for vegetations to decrease in size within the first six weeks following detection. It is however important to follow up patients with echo

detectable vegetations because an eventual decrease in size is indicative of successful therapy.

Echocardiographically, vegetations are usually seen as fuzzy, mobile echoes attached or in close proximity to the valve leaflets. In most cases the valve itself will be abnormal and occasionally, of course, prosthetic. New, active vegetations tend to have a soft, dark appearance with a gray level similar to that of myocardial tissue. Healed vegetations containing fibrous tissue tend to appear much brighter.

Figure 9.1 is an M-Mode echo of a bicuspid aortic valve with a vegetation attached. In this case, the vegetation was due to a gonococcal organism and the abnormal eccentric closure line of the aortic valve suggested that the valve was bicuspid. During diastole the vegetation can be seen as a fuzzy, irregular echo adjoining the valve closure line. In systole, the passage of blood through the aortic valve leaflets has blown the vegetation out of the M-Mode echo beam and therefore it is only seen in diastole. Figure 9.2 shows another mobile aortic valve vegetation prolapsing into the left ventricular outflow tract during diastole.

Figure 9.3 illustrates a very rare case of endocarditis. The vegetations are on the pulmonary valve, which is most unusual, and in addition they are of fungal origin, which is also rare. This patient was on immunosuppressive therapy following a renal transplant and the infection was almost certainly acquired through a central venous line. The vegetations were extremely mobile and prolapsed in and out of the right ventricular outflow tract. Following several months of therapy, a gradual decrease in size of the two vegetations has been documented. Although these masses were clearly seen with the 2D technique, the M-Mode was not at all diagnostic and this emphasizes the important role of 2D echo in this type of pathology.

Vegetations can occur on all cardiac valves and will usually have appearances similar to those discussed above. However, it can be extremely difficult to determine the presence of vegetations on valves that are calcified or prosthetic

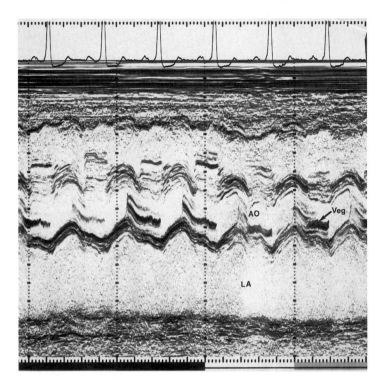

Figure 9.1   M-Mode echo of a bicuspid aortic valve with attached vegetation secondary to gonococcal endocarditis. The vegetation is seen as a fuzzy echo in diastole. During systole it is blown clear of the valve leaflets by the passage of blood through the aortic orifice.

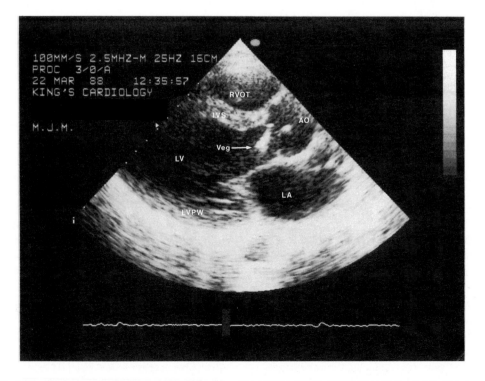

Figure 9.2   Diastolic long axis image in a patient with bacterial endocarditis. A large (2 cm) mobile vegetation is seen attached to the valve leaflets and is prolapsing into the left ventricular outflow tract.

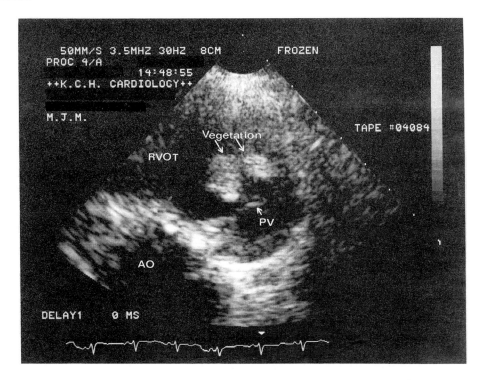

Figure 9.3 A short axis view of the aorta and right ventricular outflow tract in a patient with fungal infection of the pulmonary valve. The two globular masses, each approximately 1 cm in diameter, are attached to the pulmonary valve leaflets and during diastole are positioned within the right ventricular outflow tract. These vegetations are again highly mobile and during systole moved into the pulmonary artery.

(especially if image quality is suboptimal) since the strong echoes generated by those structures will usually mask the more delicate vegetation echoes.

Intracardiac thrombi

The recognition of thrombus within the heart is a relatively new application of echocardiography, especially with the advent of transesophageal imaging. Fortunately, even in the early stages of thrombus formation, the acoustic density changes enough for it to be visualized echocardiographically. Usually it appears as a luminous mass with much brighter echoes than the surrounding myocardium and blood.

Thrombus is most commonly seen in the left ventricle, associated with a wall motion abnormality (often due to infarction). In addition, it is usually present in the left ventricular apex where stasis of blood is most likely to occur.

It is now well recognized that mobile thrombi, frequently exposed on at least three sides, are most at risk of embolization. However, this type of echo appearance is not necessarily an indication for anticoagulation since erosion of the

thrombus attachment to the chamber wall may premeditate an embolic event.

Figure 9.4 represents a typical example of an apical, left ventricular, mobile thrombus. This apical four chamber view of a patient with poor left ventricular function due to myocarditis shows a bright spherical mass within the left ventricular apex. It had the typical appearance of thrombus. On the real-time 2D echo the mass was also seen to be very mobile and attached by a thin stalk to the left ventricular apex. Three days following commencement of anticoagulation therapy, the patient suffered an embolus to the right femoral artery. Repeat echocardiography showed a much smaller and hardly visible thrombus, presumably due to detachment and embolization of part of its structure.

Laminated thrombus which lines the endocardial wall and is not pedunculated has a lower risk of embolization. An example of this type of thrombus is illustrated in Figure 9.5. This 2D apical long axis view shows a bright mass attached to and filling the left ventricular apex. The adjoining area of myocardium was akinetic due to myocardial infarction and the mass was presumed thrombus. It was not mobile and was exposed only on one side. Subsequent cardiac catheterization and left ventricular angiography was also highly suggestive of organized immobile thrombus in the left ventricu-

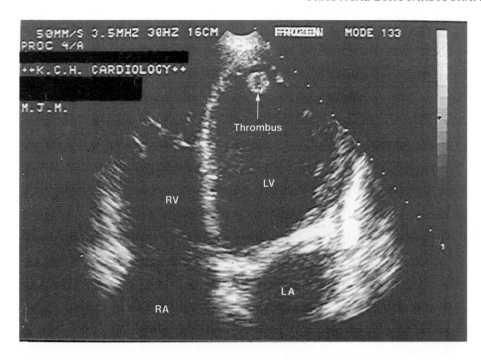

Figure 9.4 A small (1 cm), spherical thrombus is seen in the apex of the left ventricle in this apical four chamber view. The patient was suffering from acute myocarditis and consequently had very poor left ventricular function. The thrombus was mobile and embolized to the right femoral artery following commencement of anticoagulation therapy.

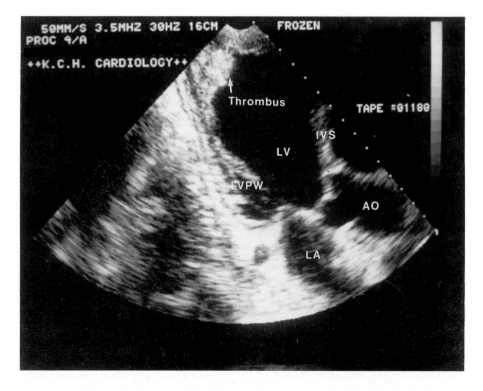

Figure 9.5 Apical long axis view in a patient with previous myocardial infarction and an aneurysmal left ventricular apex. A bright, immobile mass is seen occupying the apex and consists of laminated thrombus. The fact that this thrombus was not moving and was only exposed on one side suggests that it is at reduced risk of embolization when compared with the thrombus illustrated in Figure 9.6.

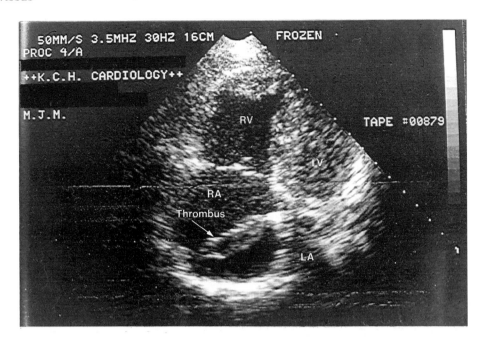

Figure 9.6 Modified apical four chamber view showing mainly the right ventricle and right atrium. Within the right atrium a tubular mass is seen, which on real-time images was freely mobile. This was presumed to be thrombus and subsequently confirmed as an embolized thrombotic venous cast.

lar apex. However, several studies have now confirmed that 2D echocardiography is more sensitive than angiography in detecting thrombus.

Intracardiac thrombus may occasionally be seen in any of the remaining cardiac chambers. It is usually difficult to detect in the right ventricle because of the heavy trabeculation within that chamber. It can be seen in the left atrium, especially in patients with mitral stenosis, and very rarely it can occur in the right atrium. Unfortunately, the left atrial appendage is not visualized using conventional echo, and it appears that this structure is an extremely common site for thrombus formation.

Right atrial thrombus may be seen in patients who have suffered pulmonary embolism. An example is illustrated in Figure 9.6. Within the right atrium a tubular mass is visible, approximately 1 cm in diameter and 4–5 cm in length. On the real-time 2D echo the mass was moving freely within the right atrium and had the appearance of an embolized venous cast. Experience has demonstrated that patients with this type of echocardiographic appearance may be in imminent danger of fresh pulmonary embolism. Therefore, urgent surgery was undertaken in this case and extensive thrombus was found and removed from the right atrium and inferior vena cava. This raises the question as to whether routine echocardiography should not indeed be undertaken in all patients with suspected pulmonary embolism.

Cardiac tumors

The most common primary tumor of the adult heart is myxoma and 75% of them are found within the left atrium, usually in women. However, myxomas are rare in children; rhabdomyomas and fibromas are the most common varieties of tumor seen in pediatric cases.

The M-Mode and 2D echocardiographic appearances of left atrial myxoma are usually very dramatic but unfortunately may be indistinguishable from atrial ball valve thrombus. Classically, myxomas are pedunculated and are attached by a narrow stalk to the interatrial septum in the region of the fossa ovalis. Indeed, an important part of the echo study is to try to visualize and establish the point of attachment of the myxoma using multiple (including subcostal) 2D views.

Myxomas are frequently extremely mobile and will be carried with the diastolic flow of blood through the mitral valve leaflets until restrained by their stalk. This will normally occur in the mitral valve orifice and consequently cause significant hemodynamic obstruction to mitral valve blood flow. Therefore patients with left atrial myxoma usually have the clinical presentation of mitral stenosis and the correct diagnosis is finally established by echocardiography.

Urgent surgery, without further investigation, is then performed in most cases.

The size and mobile nature of a typical myxoma can be appreciated from the 2D images in Figure 9.7. In systole, the tumor can be seen within the left atrium and the mitral valve leaflets are closed. In the diastolic frame, the tumor is suspended in the mitral valve orifice with the valve leaflets wrapped around it. Therefore it is highly mobile, moving between the left atrium and mitral valve orifice with every cardiac cycle. The friable nature of these tumors coupled with their mobility produces a high risk of embolization.

A typical left atrial myxoma is seen in Plate 9.1. It is suspended by its narrow stalk from the forceps and the waisted region on the main body of the tumor is where the mitral valve leaflets impinged upon it during diastole.

The M-Mode appearances of left atrial myxoma are similar, in many respects, to those of rheumatic mitral valve disease. In the preoperative section of Figure 9.8, a dense mass of echoes arising from the tumor can be seen between the mitral valve leaflets in diastole. There is a small delay between the opening of the mitral valve leaflets and the appearance of the tumor echoes. This delay corresponds to the time taken for the tumor to travel through the left atrium to the mitral valve orifice and is an important distinguishing criterion between rheumatic mitral valve disease and left atrial myxoma. As shown in Figure 9.8, the mitral valve has a normal appearance following surgical removal of the tumor.

In Figure 9.9, a left atrial myosarcoma is illustrated. While this kind of tumor is extremely rare, it does have some features which are atypical for myxomas, the most important being lack of an obvious point of attachment to the interatrial septum. In addition, myxomas are classically mobile structures, whereas other tumors are often immobile, and indeed this was the case in Figure 9.9. It is important to be aware of these differences since a different surgical approach may be warranted depending upon the type of tumor present.

Intracardiac tumours have now been described in all cardiac chambers and within the myocardium itself. Echocardiography is undoubtedly the procedure of choice for establishing this type of diagnosis and frequently no further cardiological investigation is warranted. Current research into the ultrasound tissue characteristics of cardiac tumors and masses will increase the confidence of diagnosis and may provide some noninvasive histological information.

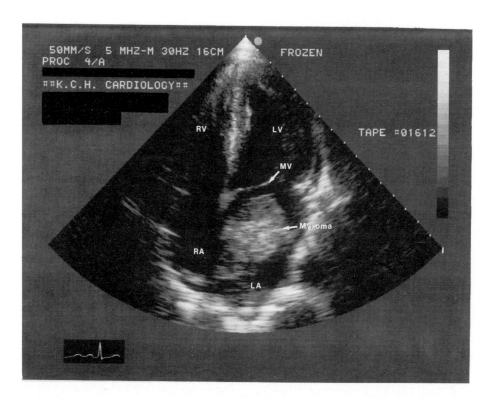

Figure 9.7a In this systolic frame a large mass is seen situated within the left atrial cavity. It is positioned adjacent to the interatrial septum and is clearly separate from the mitral valve leaflets.

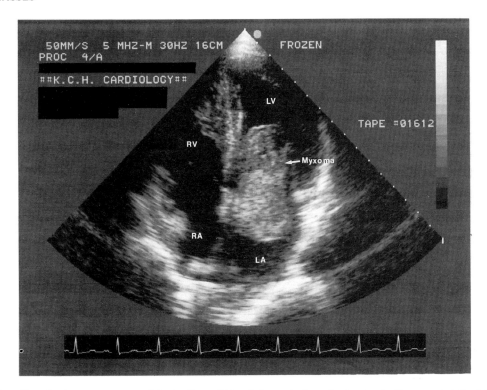

Figure 9.7b   During diastole the mass moves with the flow of blood through the mitral valve leaflets toward the left ventricle. As this image shows, the mass is suspended in diastole between the mitral valve leaflets and is held back by its attachment to the septum. It is extremely large, at approximately 7 cm in length, and has all the features of a left atrial myxoma. This was subsequently confirmed at cardiac surgery.

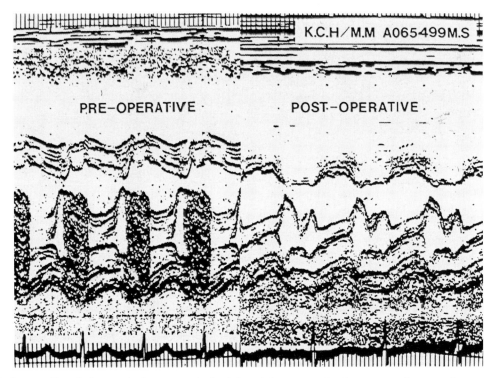

Figure 9.8   M-Mode recordings before and after removal of a left atrial myxoma. In the preoperative recording a mass of dense echoes is seen behind the mitral valve during diastole. Note that there is a slight delay between the mitral valve leaflets opening and the echoes appearing between the leaflets. This delay represents the time taken for the tumor to travel through the left atrium and arrive between the valve leaflets. Following surgical removal the classic normal mitral valve pattern is seen.

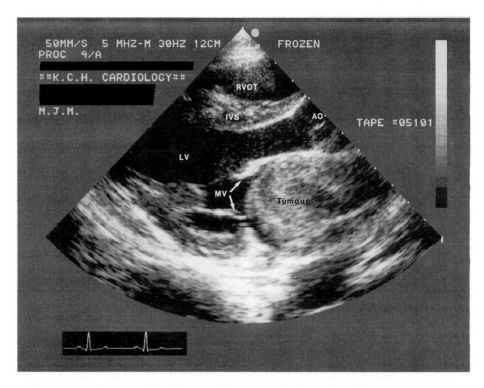

Figure 9.9a Parasternal long axis view in a patient with a large mass within the left atrium. This mass was atypical for myxoma in that it was immobile and no point of attachment to the interatrial septum could be demonstrated. Subsequent pathological examination demonstrated this to be a myosarcoma.

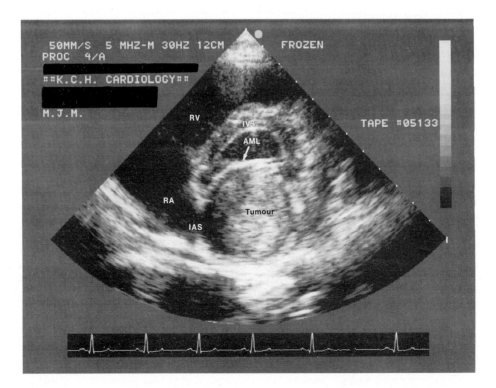

Figure 9.9b Parasternal short axis view of Figure 9.9a. In this view, a separation between the tumor and the interatrial septum can be seen. This separation was also evident in other views.

CHAPTER 10

Congenital heart disease

The development of 2D echocardiography has had a tremendous impact upon the assessment and management of patients with congenital heart disease. In young patients there is little need for coronary angiography and therefore it is frequently possible to avoid cardiac catheterization in congenital cases. Indeed, echocardiography provides information and detail of anatomy not obtainable from invasive techniques.

There are now so many applications of echocardiography in congenital heart disease that many textbooks are devoted to this single topic. This chapter will demonstrate a few of the more common congenital pathologies and the basic echo diagnostic techniques.

Technically, young children and neonates are easy to image because their lungs and ribs present less of an obstruction to ultrasound transmission than in adults. Also, it is possible to use higher frequency and therefore higher resolution transducers when examining smaller hearts. As we are all aware, patient cooperation is frequently a problem in the young and it can be difficult enough to maintain transducer contact with any part of the chest wall, let alone achieve a diagnosis from the images obtained. Hence sedation is occasionally required, both for the patient and operator! Although congenital heart disease does present in adults, it is usually picked up in earlier years. Echocardiography is mainly used to serially follow progress in the older patient.

A standardized examination and diagnostic technique are essential. Often congenital disease syndromes will consist of several associated pathologies which will require detailed individual assessment. The standard 2D parasternal and apical views are used; however, suprasternal and subcostal views are also very important.

With the transducer in a suprasternal position it is possible to image the aortic arch and its connection to the carotid and subclavian arteries as shown in Figures 2.3f and 2.7h. The presence of a patent ductus will often be seen as a vessel linking the pulmonary artery and descending aorta, opposite and slightly distal to the left subclavian artery. The suprasternal view is also essential in the diagnosis of coarctation of the aorta. Narrowing of the descending aorta distal to the subclavian artery can be seen in this condition.

Subcostal imaging is used to examine the relationship of the descending aorta, inferior vena cava, liver and atria. Connection of the anatomical right atrium to the inferior and superior venae cavae and of the left atrium to the pulmonary veins should also be established in this view.

Atrial septal defects are one of the more common congenital pathologies and are usually best imaged in the subcostal view where the atrial septum is well seen, as illustrated in Figures 10.1 and 10.2. The defect is classified as sinus venosus, coronary sinus, secundum or primum depending upon the anatomical location. The latter two are the most common and the easiest to visualize. Primum defects are situated close to the mitral and tricuspid valves and the atrioventricular ring, as shown in Figure 10.3. Secundum defects are more superior and placed in the central part of the atrial septum.

Blood flow through an atrial septal defect can occur predominantly from left to right or right to left. However, there is usually a bidirectional component, and volume overload of the right ventricle is frequently present. This will result in dilatation of the right ventricle and frequently reversed or paradoxical septal motion. An example of this is shown in Figure 10.4. Controversy exists over the exact mechanism for paradoxical septal motion. However the most likely cause is an alteration in the normal pressure relationships between the right and left ventricles. 2D echo demonstrates a marked change in right ventricular shape and size when pressure and volume overload occurs. This is often best seen in a parasternal short axis view, where dilatation of the normal crescent-shaped right ventricle causes flattening of the interventricular septum and a D-shaped left ventricular configuration as shown in Figure 10.5.

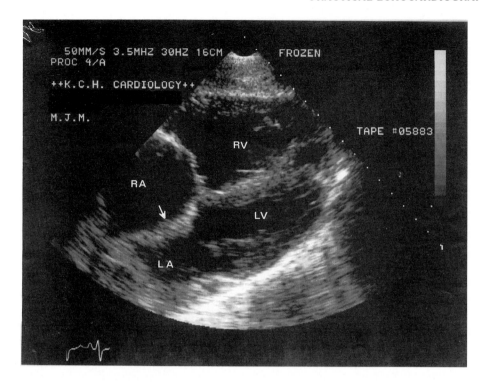

Figure 10.1 Subcostal four chamber view. The interatrial and interventricular septa are usually seen well in this view. This is because they are oriented more perpendicular rather than parallel to the interrogating ultrasound pulses from the transducer. In this case, both the septa appear intact.

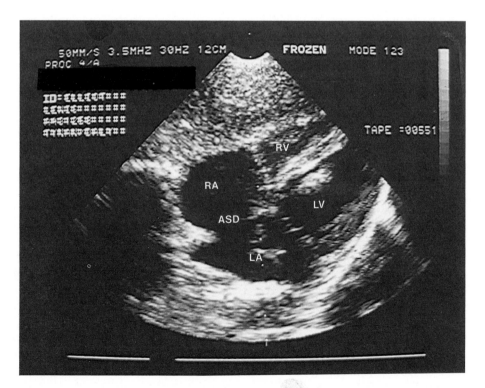

Figure 10.2 Subcostal four chamber view in a young patient with a secundum defect. A large discontinuity is seen in the mid portion of the atrial septum.

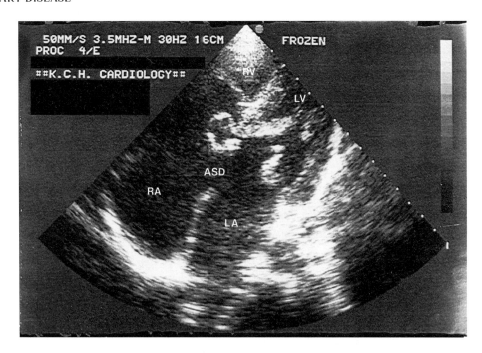

Figure 10.3 Apical four chamber view in a patient with a large primum atrial septal defect and cleft mitral valve. The right heart is very dilated, there is a large discontinuity in the atrial septum near the atrioventricular ring, and the structure and motion of the mitral valve were highly abnormal on real-time images.

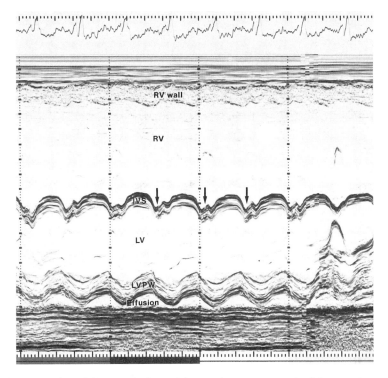

Figure 10.4 M-Mode echo demonstrating right ventricular volume and pressure overload in a patient with atrial septal defect, left-to-right shunting and pulmonary hypertension. The right ventricle is very dilated, there is right ventricular hypertrophy indicated by thickening of the right ventricular wall (anteriorly) and the septal motion is paradoxical with posterior diastolic motion (arrowed). In addition, there is a small pericardial effusion seen posteriorly.

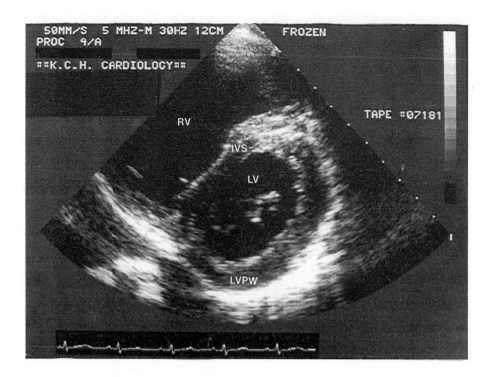

Figure 10.5 Parasternal short axis view of the right and left ventricles in a patient with right ventricular volume and pressure overload. The right ventricle is clearly grossly dilated and appears much larger than the left ventricle. In addition, the left ventricle no longer has the normal circular shape seen in this view and the interventricular septum is flattened. The left ventricle is therefore commonly described as having a D shape.

It is not always possible to directly visualize septal defects and, in addition, right ventricular volume overload may be caused by other conditions. In these cases contrast echocardiography can be used to confirm the position and site of intracardiac shunts. In this technique approximately 5 ml of agitated dextrose saline are injected rapidly into a peripheral vein. If a left arm vein is used the technique can also diagnose left-sided superior vena cava. It appears that, during the rapid injection, microcavitation occurs at the needle tip and microbubbles are brought out of solution in the injectate. These microbubbles are carried with the venous circulation through the right heart and into the lungs. In the lungs the bubbles are absorbed because they are too large to pass through the pulmonary capillary bed into the left heart. The microbubbles are very strong reflectors of ultrasound and are visualized in the right heart on M-Mode or 2D echo performed at the same time as the injection. An example is shown in Figure 10.6; as this is a normal study no bubbles are seen in the left heart. If there is a right-to-left or bidirectional shunt at either atrial or ventricular septal level, then bubbles will be seen in the left atrium and/or ventricle as shown in Figure 10.7.

If the shunt is just left to right then a negative contrast effect can often be seen on the 2D echo. Normally the bub-

bles will completely fill and opacify the right atrium and ventricle. In the region of a left-to-right shunt there may be an area of unopacified blood that can be seen on the 2D echo. Contrast echocardiography appears to be quite a safe procedure and can even be performed in neonates. In these cases it is usually possible to use the patient's own agitated blood as injectate. Doppler echocardiography (especially with color flow mapping) can be used to detect turbulent flow through shunts and has reduced the need for contrast techniques.

Defects in the ventricular septum are detected using similar techniques to those described for atrial septal defects, i.e. a combination of 2D imaging, contrast and Doppler echo. Ventricular defects are also classified in a way dependent upon their anatomical location. It is therefore very important to use all available views to obtain exact positioning of the defect, which appears as a hole or discontinuity in the septum. Subarterial defects are seen in the muscular outlet portion of the septum below the aortic and pulmonary valve rings. Perimembranous defects are in the fibrous portion of the septum attached to the aortic root and usually extend into the muscular septum. Muscular defects are by definition entirely contained by the muscular septum, may be multiple and can vary considerably in their position. Mus-

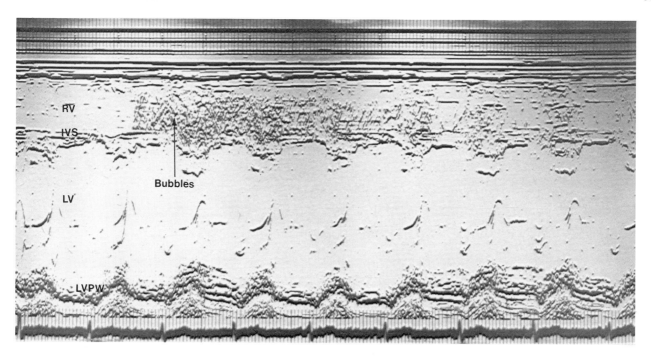

Figure 10.6 Normal M-Mode contrast echocardiogram. Microbubbles are seen entering the right ventricle; however no opacification of the left heart is visualized.

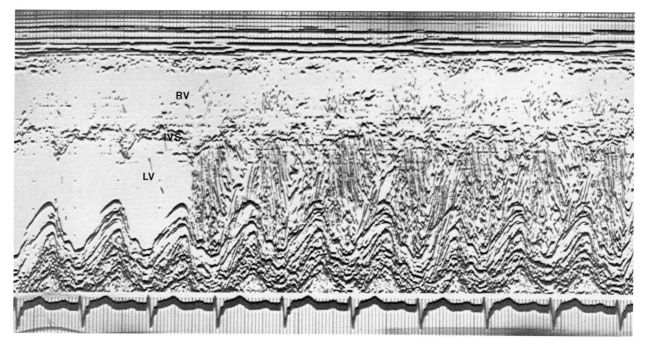

Figure 10.7 M-Mode contrast echocardiogram in a patient with an atrial septal defect and right-to-left shunting. Microbubbles are seen within the right ventricle and almost simultaneously appear within the left ventricle. In fact, the left ventricle appears to opacify more intensely than the right.

cular defects are usually the most difficult type to directly visualize. An example of a muscular defect is seen in Figure 10.8a and of a perimembranous defect in Figure 10.8b.

Since apparent defects in both the atrial and ventricular septa may be artefactually produced, it is important to confirm the diagnosis utilizing as many views as possible.

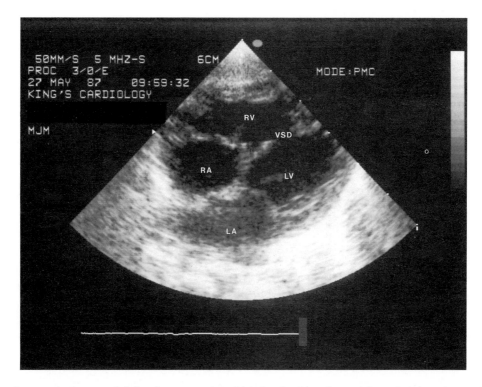

Figure 10.8a Muscular ventricular septal defect in a seven-day-old baby. In this subcostal four chamber view, a discontinuity is seen in the mid portion of the muscular septum. Confirmation of flow through this defect was obtained using Doppler.

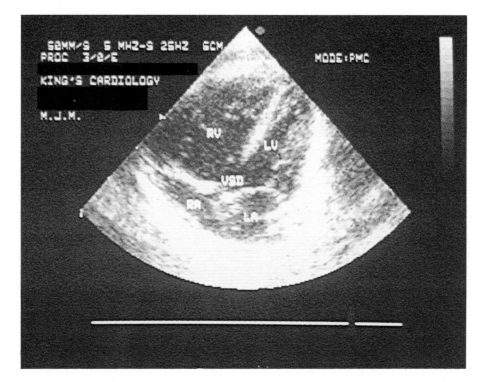

Figure 10.8b In this subcostal four chamber view a perimembranous ventricular septal defect is seen. The large septal discontinuity is positioned close to the atrioventricular ring in the membranous portion of the inflow septum. The right ventricle is significantly dilated and Doppler studies confirmed left-to-right shunting through this defect.

Atrioventricular septal defects are, as the name suggests, a combination of both atrial and ventricular septal defects. These are often associated with abnormalities of the tricuspid and mitral valves which can vary in severity and may include a common atrioventricular leaflet. An example of an atrioventricular defect and transposition is shown in Figure 10.9.

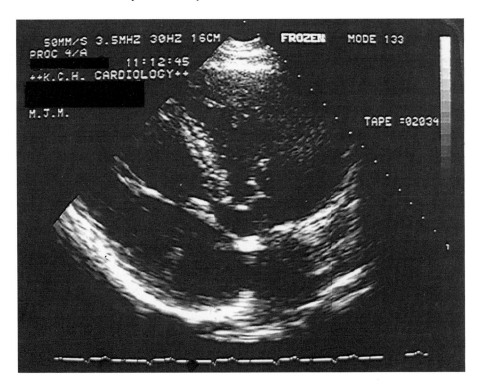

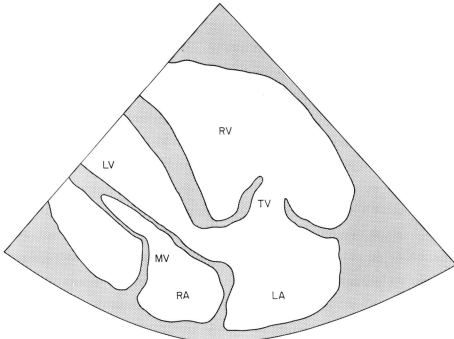

Figure 10.9 An apical four chamber view in a patient with an atrioventricular defect and transposition. The right ventricle is identified by the more apical septal insertion of the tricuspid valve. Standard imaging and contrast studies confirmed the position of the right atrium. The large defect is seen around the atrioventricular valves.

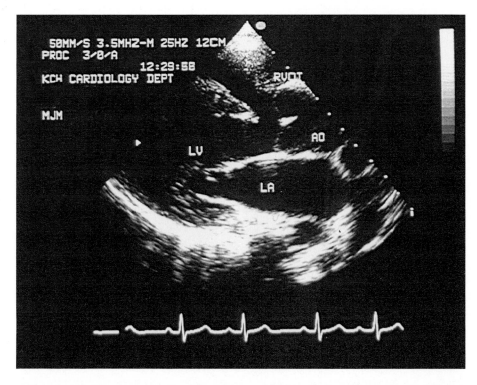

Figure 10.10 Parasternal long axis view in a patient with tetralogy of Fallot. The aortic root is very dilated and overrides a large perimembranous ventricular septal defect. Other views and Doppler studies confirmed the remaining anatomical abnormalities associated with this syndrome.

In any examination where congenital pathology is suspected, it is of course very important to establish the integrity of all anatomical connections. In other words, is the heart plumbed correctly? This should be established in a sequential manner starting with identification of vena cava and pulmonary vein attachments to the right and left atrium respectively. The next stage is to verify the relationship of the ventricles to the atria. Are both ventricles present, or is one absent or very small, i.e. hypoplastic? Both atrioventricular valves should be visualized, and therefore the presence of tricuspid or mitral atresia can be identified.

The tricuspid valve is always attached to the right ventricle. It can be identified by the presence of three leaflets and the fact that it is inserted into the ventricular septum nearer the apex than the mitral valve. The apical or subcostal four chamber are the easiest views to identify this on (see Chapter 2, Figures 2.7f and g). The right ventricle can therefore be distinguished by its attachment to the tricuspid valve. It also has more trabeculae than the left ventricle and therefore has an irregular endocardial surface which may be seen on the 2D echo. If the tricuspid valve is seen very near the apex of an apparently small right ventricle then the diagnosis of Ebstein's anomaly must be considered.

Discordant connections between the right atrium and ventricle and also the left atrium and ventricle will be present in the various forms of transposition. There is invariably an intracardiac shunt at either atrial or ventricular level also present in these conditions.

The sequential examination technique should then be continued to verify the integrity of the aortic and pulmonary artery connections to the functional left and right ventricles respectively. The aorta is identified as the vessel which courses superiorly into the aortic arch. The subclavian and carotid arteries can be seen arising from the arch. The right ventricular outflow tract and pulmonary artery wrap around the aortic root, and descend posteriorly before bifurcating into the right and left branches. This is usually easily seen on 2D imaging.

The presence of both the aorta and the pulmonary artery must be verified and therefore atresia of either of these vessels excluded. They should both arise separately from the correct ventricles so that a double outflow ventricle, truncus arteriosus or any form of transposition is also ruled out.

As previously mentioned, many congenital cardiac pathologies consist of a number of different associated lesions. One of the most common combinations is known as tetralogy of Fallot. This is characterized by a perimembranous ventricular septal defect and a large overriding aorta, giving an appearance similiar to truncus arteriosus or double outlet right ventricle. Valvular and/or infundibular pulmonary stenosis is also present and in more severe cases there may be pulmonary atresia. An example is illustrated in Figure 10.10. It should be possible to successfully identify all these lesions even in the neonate, and many surgeons are willing to perform corrective procedures based upon an echo diagnosis.

Space restrictions unfortunately preclude any more detailed discussion of this very important, interesting and challenging aspect of echocardiography. In this chapter, I have attempted to present a simplified account of echo diagnostic techniques in some of the more common congenital pathologies. Some corrective and palliative procedures are now performed entirely under echo control, often in an incubator. These can include balloon valvotomy for the treatment of congenital valvular stenosis, and atrial septostomy when it is necessary to create an atrial septal defect.

Doppler echo has now become an important and integral part of modern echo diagnosis. Nowhere is this more true than in the assessment of congenital lesions, where the ability to supplement anatomical data with details of intracardiac hemodynamics has made a tremendous difference to the management of this type of pathology.

CHAPTER 11

Doppler echocardiography

Over the past three or four years Doppler has been routinely used in many centers as an adjunct to standard M-Mode and 2D echocardiography. In essence the technique uses the Doppler principle to examine both the direction and velocity of blood flow within the heart. This can provide precise hemodynamic data about the nature and severity of valvular and congenital lesions. Information about cardiac structure and function from the standard echo is therefore very usefully complemented by this hemodynamic data.

This chapter describes the main principles and applications of Doppler echo and color flow mapping together with practical hints on examination technique.

Basic principles

The Doppler effect was first described in 1842 by the Austrian physicist Christian Johann Doppler. He described a "change in frequency of sound, light or other waves caused by the motion of the source or the observer". A classical example of this is the apparent change in pitch of a sounding car horn as the vehicle passes an observer. As the car approaches, the horn has a higher pitch and as it moves away the pitch is lower. The difference in pitch from its real (stationary) value is dependent on the relative velocities of the car and the observer. In basic terms, the faster the car horn moves towards the observer, the more the sound waves are compressed and therefore the higher the note heard. There is a direct relationship via the Doppler formula between the relative velocity of the sound source and the alteration in pitch.

It is upon this basic principle that Doppler echocardio-

Parts of this chapter have been taken from Monaghan, M.J. and Mills, P. (1989) Doppler colour flow mapping: technology in search of an application? *British Heart Journal*, vol. 61, pp. 133–138, reproduced with permission.

graphy relies. In standard echocardiography the amplitude of the returning echoes are processed to give information about the position of the reflecting interfaces, i.e. heart muscle and valves etc. (see Chapter 1). When Doppler is being performed, the returning echoes are processed in a different way to examine any changes in ultrasound frequency between the transmitted and received sound waves. These frequency shifts would be caused by moving interfaces in the sound beam path. In this case the interfaces we are interested in are the red blood cells so that we obtain blood flow information. Other moving interfaces such as valves will also cause a "Doppler shift" but this lower velocity information is largely filtered out by the instrument.

There are several Doppler techniques currently used for examining cardiac blood flow. They have a variety of advantages and disadvantages. Most instruments have the ability to perform both continuous and pulsed wave Doppler. These are the most common techniques. Color flow mapping is the latest Doppler modality and is described towards the end of this chapter.

Figures 11.1 and 11.2 illustrate the basic principles of continuous and pulsed wave Doppler respectively. It is important to remember that the shift in frequency of the sound waves is dependent upon the velocity of the red blood cells relative to the transducer that is transmitting and receiving the sound waves. Therefore, the position of the transducer is usually arranged so that the direction of blood flow (in the area of interest) is parallel to the plane of the sound waves. If there is an angle between the direction of the sound pulses and the blood flow, then absolute measurement of blood velocity cannot be made without some correction. This can itself introduce errors. It is for this reason that the cardiac apex is usually the most useful transducer position to use during a Doppler examination of left heart blood flow. As shown in Figures 11.1 and 11.2, blood flow into the left ventricle through the mitral valve and out through the aorta occurs in a plane which is more or less parallel to the sound

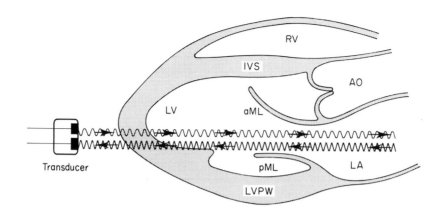

Figure 11.1 Diagram of continuous-wave Doppler principles. The transducer is positioned over the apex and directed so that sound travels through the mitral valve. Both transmitted and reflected/received sound wave beams are shown. Since the diagram represents diastole, flow through the mitral valve is toward the transducer and the reflected sound waves are shifted upwards in frequency. It is important to remember, however, that all blood velocities occurring down the beam path are detected and displayed simultaneously.

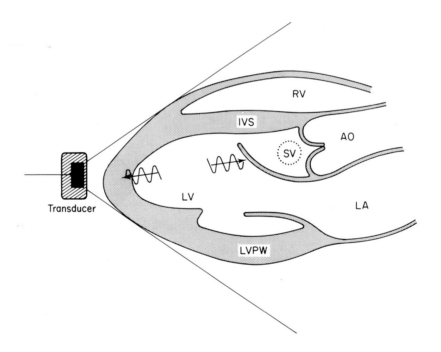

Figure 11.2 Diagram illustrating pulsed Doppler examination. The transducer is positioned over the cardiac apex and the sample volume position is selected in the left ventricular outflow tract. A transmitted sound pulse (fixed frequency) traveling toward the sample volume and a reflected sound pulse (shifted frequency) returning are shown. If no flow occurred in the sample volume then transmitted and received frequencies would be the same. The diagram represents diastole and if the returning sound had been of a higher frequency it would have indicated blood flow toward the transducer. This would probably be due to aortic regurgitation.

waves coming from the transducer positioned over the cardiac apex.

Other transducer positions would also routinely be used during a Doppler examination. These would depend upon the type and site of blood flow being studied (see Table 11.1).

From a patient's point of view, having a Doppler examination is very similar to a standard echo, with the exception that the shift in Doppler frequency is often output both to the display screen and as an audio signal to guide the operator. These noises can sound somewhat alarming and have been likened to those produced by "space invader" games.

Table 11.1

Site of interest	Doppler transducer position
Aortic valve	Apex, suprasternal, right parasternal
Ascending aorta	Apex, suprasternal
Descending aorta	Suprasternal
Mitral valve	Apex
Tricuspid valve	Apex, parasternal, midprecordial
Pulmonary valve	Parasternal, midprecordial, subcostal
Pulmonary artery	Parasternal, midprecordial, subcostal

In fact performing a Doppler examination is probably more fun but also more difficult than playing space invaders!

In Figure 11.1, a continuous wave transducer is shown positioned over the cardiac apex so that the sound waves are directed through the left ventricle, mitral valve and left atrium. As shown, the continuous wave transducer has two elements, one of which continuously transmits sound of a particular frequency (often around 2 MHz) and the other element detects the returning sound waves which will vary in frequency depending upon the velocity of the blood down the sound path. The frequency of the returning sound waves is analyzed by the instrument and the Doppler shift is output as an audio signal and also converted into velocity which is displayed in graphical format. The latter is illustrated in Figure 11.3 and is a graph of velocity against time with a simultaneous ECG which is important for timing the blood flow. Velocities above the zero line represent flow towards the transducer and below the line flow away from the transducer. Blood velocities down the entire continuous wave path are detected and displayed by this technique. Therefore both the low blood velocities proximal to a stenotic lesion and the high velocities distal to it will be superimposed on the display. This type of Doppler display is called "spectral" because variations in gray scale on the recording are used to illustrate changes in intensity of the received Doppler signal. Hence they represent the relative number of red blood cells (within the Doppler beam) travelling at each velocity and direction. This means, for example, in Figure 11.3 that the large number of blood cells travelling together at a relatively low velocity in the left ventricular outflow tract

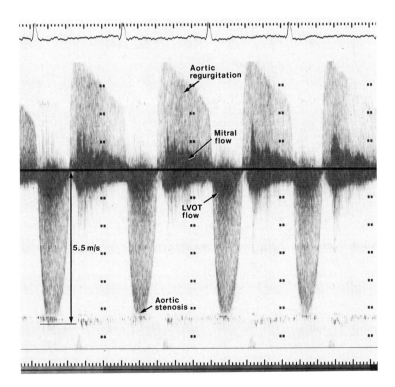

Figure 11.3 Continuous wave Doppler recording from the apex in a patient with severe aortic stenosis and regurgitation. The continuous wave Doppler beam is directed through the left ventricular outflow tract and aortic valve. In systole a high velocity (5.5 m/s) jet is seen going through the valve. Since the jet is moving away from the transducer it is displayed below the zero line, whereas in diastole high velocity flow (peak 4 m/s) is seen above the zero line traveling toward the transducer and is due to aortic regurgitation. The spectral display indicates low velocity flow during systole in the left ventricular outflow tract, shown by the darker portion of the gray scale recording. During diastole, the low velocity, dark signals are from mitral inflow. Therefore, with good spectral display it is frequently possible to appreciate blood flows of different velocities occurring in different parts of the ventricle when they are superimposed upon the continuous wave recording.

is seen as a dense, dark signal, whereas above the stenotic valve the velocity of the blood cells is increased and they are more dispersed so that a lighter and higher velocity signal is superimposed. Good spectral Doppler recordings should allow one to appreciate the relative quantities of blood cells travelling at each velocity. In addition, they should be especially sensitive to weak jets through stenotic valves which are likely to occur at high velocities.

Figure 11.2 is used to illustrate the principle of pulsed Doppler. This technique is usually performed with a standard 2D transducer and the outer margins of the imaging sector are shown in the figure. With pulsed Doppler it is possible to examine blood flow at any one particular point in the imaging plane. A sample volume position is selected on the 2D image, usually with the assistance of a joystick or track-ball. In Figure 11.2 the sample volume is shown placed immediately beneath the aortic valve in the left ventricular outflow tract. When the pulsed Doppler section of the instrument is activated, the ultrasound pulses are directed down a path from the transducer so that they pass through the sample volume. The instrument knows where the sample volume is. Therefore, it is able to calculate exactly how long it will take for a transmitted sound pulse

to travel to and be reflected off the red blood cells in the sample volume, and travel back to the transducer. The receiver portion of the instrument is then only listening at the time when sound from the sample volume will be returning. As soon as it has been received, the next pulse is transmitted and so on. In this way, only blood velocity information at a specific point in the heart is analyzed, unlike the continuous wave technique, which displays all velocities down the sound beam simultaneously. An example of pulsed Doppler recording in the left ventricular outflow tract is seen in Figure 11.4.

Spectral Doppler display is also important in pulsed Doppler. If blood flow within the sample volume is laminar, then all the blood cells should be moving with similar velocity and direction. Therefore, the velocity recording profile should be narrow, indicating that all the cells are moving together. However, if blood flow in and around the sample volume is turbulent then the cells will be moving with varying direction and velocity. "Spectral broadening" will then be seen on the recordings and the velocity flow profile will be wide and possibly filled in.

Both continuous and pulsed techniques have different advantages and disadvantages. They essentially complement

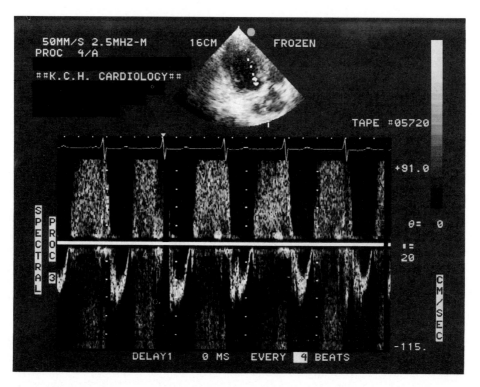

Figure 11.4 Pulsed wave Doppler recording from the left ventricular outflow tract obtained using an apical long axis view. In systole, laminar low velocity flow is seen moving away from the transducer, whereas in diastole a high velocity, aliased (see text) signal is recorded. The signal should not be present in a normal subject and is due to aortic regurgitation. In order to obtain an indication of the size and significance of the regurgitant jet the sample volume may be moved throughout the ventricle and the spatial extent of the turbulent signal documented.

each other and provide different types of information. Because continuous wave Doppler uses a specialized transducer, it is more sensitive than pulsed and it also has a very high limit on the maximum blood velocity that can be detected. One of the disadvantages is that, unlike pulsed Doppler, there is not usually an image to guide and show the direction of the continuous wave beam. This disadvantage can be overcome to a certain extent by using an imaging transducer with continuous wave transducer elements mounted at one side. Alternatively, the imaging elements themselves may be used to create a line of continuous wave Doppler that may be varied in direction. A marking line is then displayed on the 2D image to illustrate the direction of the continuous wave Doppler. However, a combined imaging and continuous wave transducer is not as sensitive as a separate, stand-alone Doppler transducer and it is usually worth persevering with the latter.

Most novices find pulsed Doppler easier to use than continuous wave because the exact position of Doppler sampling can be seen and guided by the 2D image. However, there are technical conflicts between imaging and Doppler requirements in a transducer. Since pulsed Doppler is normally performed with an imaging transducer, the Doppler is less sensitive and small jets are difficult to detect. Red blood cells act as scatterers rather than reflectors of sound waves and therefore the intensity of the returning sound waves is very low and transducer sensitivity is important. There is another very important technical limitation with pulsed Doppler that relates to the fact that velocities are being sampled by the pulses rather than continuously detected. This effectively limits the maximum velocity that can be detected by pulsed Doppler and is dependent on both the frequency of the transducer and also the depth of the sample volume. A physical term called the "Nyquist limit" defines this maximum detectable frequency shift and hence velocity. If the velocity of blood in the sample volume relative to the transducer exceeds the maximum detectable velocity then a phenomenon known as aliasing occurs. Here, the high velocity signal goes off the scale of the display and appears as a velocity signal in the opposite direction. At first this can appear quite confusing and usually prevents the peak velocity from actually being measured. Very often, aliasing will occur to such an extent that the high velocity signal is in fact "wrapped around" the display several times and appears as a dense band of signals in both the positive and negative parts of the velocity display.

This aliasing phenomenon is analogous to the effect seen in old movies such as Westerns where a rotating stagecoach wheel is being filmed using a camera with a relatively slow frame rate. The rotating wheel is being effectively sampled by the frame rate of the camera in the same way that pulsed Doppler is sampling the Doppler frequency shift. When the wheel is rotating at a rate which is much lower than the camera frame rate then its direction and velocity can be seen. As the wheel increases in speed it will reach a point when the rotation rate is half the camera frame rate. This is the Nyquist limit and the direction of wheel rotation can no longer be appreciated. As the rotation rate increases beyond the Nyquist limit, the wheel appears to be going backwards and this is the same as aliasing. When the rotation rate equals the frame rate the wheel appears stationary because it will be in the same relative position every time it is recorded on film. Therefore in order to faithfully record the direction and velocity of blood flow we must operate below the Nyquist limit. This limit is dependent on two important factors. The first of these is the pulse repetition rate of the Doppler (how often we are sampling the frequency shift); this rate is higher when the sample volume is near the transducer and the sound does not have so far to travel. The Nyquist limit is also dependent on the frequency of the transducer, since it is around this central transmitted frequency that the Doppler shift occurs. Therefore, the velocity at which aliasing occurs will be higher for low frequency transducers with near sample volumes.

Normal examination

Table 11.1 has illustrated the general Doppler transducer positions for recording intracardiac flow. Precise transducer positioning is usually achieved by using the 2D image to guide and orient the Doppler beam direction (and sample volume) with respect to anatomical structures. Wherever possible, it is important to try to align the Doppler beam direction so that it is likely to be parallel with flow and hence minimize any velocity errors. The direction of abnormal flow jets is not always predictable and color flow mapping (discussed later) can be very helpful in this context. However, when using conventional Doppler, "fine tuning" of the beam position and direction should be achieved by looking for the point of highest velocity with the strongest spectral and audio signal.

Most people find it easier to commence a Doppler examination using pulsed wave, since this is normally guided by the image. Peak flows through all the valves, in the aorta and in the pulmonary artery should be recorded. In addition, the sample volume should be moved around behind each valve to pick up any regurgitant jets. Continuous wave recordings of flow through every valve should also be attempted, since this technique is more sensitive than pulsed Doppler and may record small, previously undetected jets. Continuous wave will also allow higher velocities to be recorded, without aliasing, than is possible using pulsed Doppler.

Table 11.2 shows the normal peak flow velocities for adults and children. Most pulsed wave Doppler systems should be capable of recording these velocities without aliasing.

Table 11.2 Maximal Doppler velocities in normal individuals (m/s)

	Children	Adults
Mitral flow	1.00 (0.8–1.3)	0.90 (0.6–1.3)
Tricuspid flow	0.60 (0.5–0.8)	0.50 (0.3–0.7)
Pulmonary artery	0.90 (0.7–1.1)	0.75 (0.6–0.9)
Left ventricle	1.00 (0.7–1.2)	0.90 (0.7–1.1)
Aorta	1.50 (1.2–1.8)	1.35 (1.0–1.7)

(From L. Hatle and B. Anglesen *Doppler Ultrasound in Cardiology*, p 72, Lea & Febiger.)

When examining a Doppler recording it is often helpful to go through the following checklist of points. After a time your eye will pattern-recognize abnormal flow configurations.

1. Is pulsed or continuous wave Doppler used?
2. What is the presumed beam direction/sampling site?
3. Does the general flow profile confirm this?
4. Is flow moving in the right direction at the right time (use ECG)?
5. Are unexpected flows present at the wrong time (use ECG)?
6. Is the signal aliasing (on pulsed Doppler)?
7. Is the flow profile strong and well defined suggesting parallel alignment?
8. Are flow velocities within the normal range?

This is by no means an exhaustive list; however, it does provide a starting point for qualitative analysis of Doppler recordings. More specific points will be highlighted in the following sections on abnormal flow patterns.

Valvular stenosis

As blood passes through any stenotic valve, its velocity will increase. There is a direct relationship between the velocity of blood through an obstruction and the pressure gradient generated across it. This relationship was first described by the Dutch physicist Daniel Bernouilli. His equation relating fluid velocity and pressure gradient is in fact extremely complicated. Fortunately, however, it can be dramatically simplified, and its application to measurement of pressure gradients across stenotic valves was first described by Holen and Hatle in 1976. The modified Bernouilli equation is given as:

$$P_1 - P_2 = 4(V_2^2 - V_1^2)$$

where $P_1 - P_2$ = the pressure gradient in mmHg
V_2 = the peak velocity distal to the obstruction
V_1 = the peak velocity proximal to the obstruction

In most situations the velocity proximal to the valve is below 1.5 m/s and its effect is negligible and so it may be ignored. The simplified Bernouilli equation is then:

$$P_1 - P_2 = 4V^2$$

where V = the peak blood velocity measured through the valve

Very often the peak velocity will be above the Nyquist limit for pulsed Doppler examination and aliasing will result. This may mean that it is impossible to measure the peak velocity using pulsed Doppler. If the velocity is only just above the Nyquist limit then shifting the zero baseline (or using the spectral unwrapping feature on some instruments) will allow measurement of peak velocity.

Generally, however, it is necessary to use continuous wave Doppler to record the high velocities through stenotic valves. Since this technique is also more sensitive than pulsed wave it also reduces the likelihood of missing the peak velocity.

As there is a squared relationship between the velocity and gradient, it is imperative that the velocity measurement should be as accurate as possible. Therefore, every attempt should be made to limit the angle of incidence between the Doppler beam and jet direction. In addition, where possible, recordings should be taken from several positions (and the highest velocity analyzed), and measurements should only be made from recordings where the velocity profile is clearly defined. There have been many studies demonstrating an excellent correlation between Doppler estimates of pressure gradients and those obtained using simultaneous recordings with pressure tip catheters. The correlation is less excellent if comparisons are not simultaneous and are made with fluid-filled catheters, often using a pressure withdrawal across the valve or pulmonary wedge as an estimate of left atrial pressure. In these cases, it is likely that the errors lie with the catheter rather than the Doppler gradient measurements!

Measurements of mean pressure gradient may be made by calculating the gradient at multiple points during the flow profile and deriving a mean. Because of the squared relationship between velocity and gradient, it is not possible to simply calculate a mean velocity and derive the gradient from that. Most Doppler instruments contain analysis software (also available as a separate package) which makes calculation of mean gradients etc. much simpler and less tedious than manual methods.

Aortic stenosis

Since pulsed Doppler aliases at comparatively low velocities, it is of little use in the evaluation of aortic stenosis where even a trivial gradient will generate velocities of over 2 m/s.

In most patients, the best peak aortic valve velocities will be recorded with the transducer situated at the cardiac apex, when flow through the valve in systole will be seen below the zero line, since it is moving away from the transducer. Using conventional 2D imaging, the best continuous wave transducer position can be selected so that the Doppler beam can be directed through the left ventricle, outflow tract and aortic valve in a direction that is likely to be parallel to flow. It is usually easier to visualize beam alignment with an apical long axis view. If a separate Doppler transducer is being used, it should be substituted for the imaging probe and directed so that the beam should point toward the aortic valve. Minor adjustment to the Doppler transducer position and angulation are made by reference to both the audio and spectral signals, so that the highest velocity and cleanest profile is recorded.

Since the continuous wave technique records all blood velocities within the beam, it is quite possible that, in some patients, diastolic left ventricle inflow velocities will be recorded together with aortic outflow. However, if a strong left ventricle inflow signal is seen, then this usually means that the Doppler beam requires a more medial and anterior angulation toward the aortic valve. The aortic valve is some distance from the transducer at the apex and therefore small changes in transducer direction will move the Doppler beam quite considerably at valve level. It is very useful to listen to the Doppler audio signal when searching for a small high velocity jet, since the high-pitched Doppler audio signal is usually audible before it is seen in the spectral display. This indicates that the Doppler beam is almost aligned.

In Figure 11.3 a continuous wave Doppler recording of aortic stenosis is seen. The aortic systolic flow profile is clearly defined with a "peaked" shape and relatively short duration. This is a high quality spectral recording and the darker, lower velocities from blood flow in the outflow tract proximal to the valve can be seen. Since this proximal flow is below 1.5 m/s it can be ignored and the simplified Bernouilli equation used to calculate the peak gradient. In patients with significant aortic regurgitation, the subaortic velocity may be elevated and the standard Bernouilli calculation (as shown above) must be utilized. Pulsed Doppler may be used to record the subaortic velocity if it cannot be seen clearly on continuous wave.

The direction of an aortic stenotic jet can be very eccentric and it may be that, despite appearances to the contrary, an apical transducer may not provide best beam alignment and so an artificially low velocity is recorded. Therefore it is important that the other examination positions, as shown in Table 11.1, are used and the highest resultant velocity used to calculate peak gradient. The right parasternal position is often possible in patients with aortic stenosis because of poststenotic aortic dilatation and some aortic unfolding. Patients should lie on their right side (almost leaning forward) and the 2D imaging transducer may be moved along the right parasternal edge to find the ascending aorta and aortic root. The continuous wave transducer is then positioned accordingly and the Doppler beam directed under the sternum toward the aortic valve. Again, fine tuning of the transducer position and angulation will inevitably be required to record the highest and best Doppler profile. When using this transducer position, aortic systolic flow will be directed up toward the transducer and will therefore be seen above the Doppler zero line, as shown in Figure 11.5.

It is important to remember that when the results of Doppler estimation of aortic valve gradient are compared with those obtained nonsimultaneously with fluid-filled catheters at cardiac catheterization, Doppler measures the peak instantaneous gradient which is different and usually higher than the peak-to-peak gradient commonly measured at catheterization. In addition, it is worth noting that since peak aortic and peak left ventricular pressure points (in aortic stenosis) occur at different times during systole, the peak-to-peak gradient is actually nonphysiological. These points are illustrated in Figure 11.6.

Doppler may be used to calculate the aortic valve area by a number of different methods. The simplest technique is to utilize the continuity equation which works on the premise that, at any point in a closed system, the product of flow velocity and cross-sectional area are the same. When this is applied to flow in the left ventricular outflow tract and aortic valve, the subaortic velocity multiplied by the subaortic cross-sectional area will equal the aortic valve velocity multiplied by the aortic valve area. Figure 11.7 is a diagrammatic illustration of the application of the continuity equation through a stenotic aortic valve. V_1 (the velocity in the left ventricular outflow tract) may be measured using pulsed Doppler, or on continuous wave Doppler when the darker spectral flow profile of the subvalvar velocities is easily identified. The high velocity through the stenotic valve (V_2) will need to be measured using continuous wave Doppler because aliasing will almost certainly occur on pulsed Doppler. Originally mean velocities were used in the continuity equation. However, it has now been shown that it is unnecessary to calculate mean velocities and that the easily measured peak velocities will suffice. The subaortic area is calculated from the diameter (measured on 2D echo as in Figure 11.32), so that:

$$\text{Aortic valve area (cm}^2) = \frac{V_1 \times A_1}{V_2}$$

where V_1 = subaortic peak velocity (cm/s)
A_1 = subaortic area: $\pi \times (\text{diameter}/2)^2$
V_2 = aortic peak velocity (cm/s)

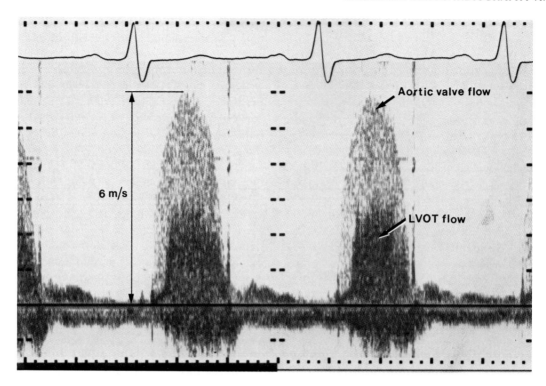

Figure 11.5 Continuous wave Doppler recording of aortic valve flow from the right parasternal edge. In this patient with aortic stenosis, high velocity flow (6 m/s) is seen coming toward the transducer. The spectral recording demonstrates that the flow within the left ventricular outflow tract (the darker signal) has a peak velocity of approximately 3 m/s and therefore cannot be ignored. In this case, the conventional Bernouilli equation must be used so that the subvalvular velocity is included in the calculation of the pressure gradient.

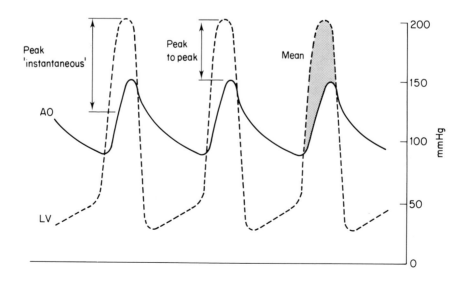

Figure 11.6 Diagrammatic representation of simultaneous aortic and left ventricular pressure tracings in a patient with aortic stenosis. The peak instantaneous gradient measured by Doppler is larger than the peak to peak gradient conventionally measured at cardiac catheterization. It can be seen that since aortic and left ventricular peak pressures occur at different times, the peak to peak gradient is in fact nonphysiological. The mean gradient, which can be calculated from the Doppler recordings, represents the average left ventricular to aortic pressure gradient during systole.

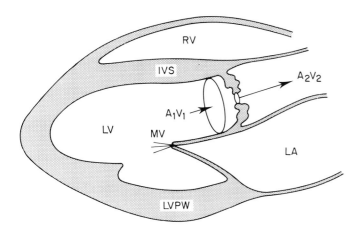

Figure 11.7 Diagram illustrating the principle of the continuity equation for calculating aortic valve area. The product of cross-sectional area and velocity in the left ventricular outflow tract should equal the product of the velocity through the valve and aortic valve area.

$$A_1 V_1 \; = \; A_2 V_2$$
$$\therefore \quad A_2 \; = \; \frac{A_1 V_1}{V_2}$$

The largest source of error in this technique lies in the calculation of subaortic area, which is derived from the diameter. However, when the continuity equation is used to study relative changes in aortic valve area following procedures such as valvuloplasty, it is particularly useful because it can be assumed that the subaortic area does not change after the procedure and so the same value may be used.

Mitral stenosis

Pressure gradients in mitral stenosis are obviously considerably lower than in aortic stenosis. Consequently, transmitral velocities may usually be recorded using pulsed Doppler without aliasing. However, the width of the pulsed Doppler sample volume is often less than that of the mitral inflow jet and hence it is possible (without careful searching) that the highest velocity point may be missed. This is less likely with continuous wave Doppler since all velocities along the beam are recorded and the beam is also wider.

Whichever Doppler technique is used, the transducer is placed at the apex so that diastolic mitral flow is directed toward the transducer and is seen above the zero line. The

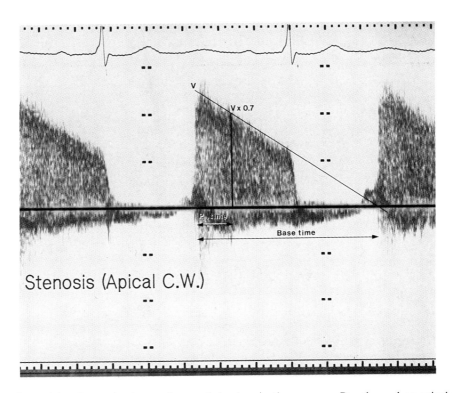

Figure 11.8 High velocity flow arising from mitral stenosis recorded using continuous wave Doppler and an apical transducer position. Flow toward the transducer is seen in diastole. It has a peak velocity of approximately 2.4 m/s and a slow rate of descent. The pressure-half-time is calculated by measuring the time taken for the peak velocity to decline to 0.7 of its original value. The mitral valve area may be empirically estimated by the formula

$$\text{Mitral valve area (cm}^2) \; = \; \frac{220}{\text{Pressure half-time}}$$

precise Doppler transducer position is selected after study of the mitral valve anatomy using apical four chamber and long axis views so that the likely mitral jet direction can be estimated. The Doppler transducer position and angulation are then adjusted accordingly, and fine tuning is achieved (as before) using the audio and spectral indicators of the highest velocity and clearest flow profile. Color flow mapping is also very useful in aligning the Doppler beam since the true jet direction is easily appreciated.

An example of continuous wave recording in mitral stenosis is shown in Figure 11.8. The entire inflow velocity profile is increased and, in addition, the rate of decline of velocity during diastole is slow, indicating reduced left ventricular filling.

The simplified Bernouilli equation may again be used to measure the mitral valve gradient at any point during diastole. Simultaneous catheter studies have also shown an excellent correlation with Doppler measurements. End-diastolic gradients are commonly quoted at cardiac catheterization and are easily measured with Doppler by utilizing the end-diastolic velocity. However, there is usually considerable beat-to-beat variability in this measurement, particularly in patients with atrial fibrillation and varying R–R intervals, so it is sensible to take an average of several gradient measurements.

Mean mitral gradients show less beat-to-beat variation and may be calculated as before by averaging measurements of gradient at multiple intervals during diastole or by using a Doppler analysis system where the whole of the mitral inflow velocity profile is traced into a computer. The latter is obviously less tedious and therefore one may be more encouraged to analyze several cardiac cycles! An example of computer derived mean mitral gradient calculation is seen in Figure 11.9.

Transvalvar pressure gradients are flow dependent and therefore any alteration in cardiac output and hence forward flow across a valve will have an effect on the pressure gradient. This is particularly true in mitral stenosis, and in many Cardiology centers the valve area (which is independent of flow) is used to grade the severity of stenosis. As described in Chapter 4, the mitral valve area may be measured by direct planimetry from 2D echo. In many patients with severe stenosis and small irregular orifices, planimetry may be difficult. Doppler can also be used to calculate mitral valve area by utilizing a pressure half-time technique that was originally conceived for cardiac catheterization. This technique has been adapted for Doppler by Hatle and colleagues. It utilizes the fact that the rate of decline of a mitral pressure gradient is directly proportional to the valve area. The rate of pressure decline is in fact expressed

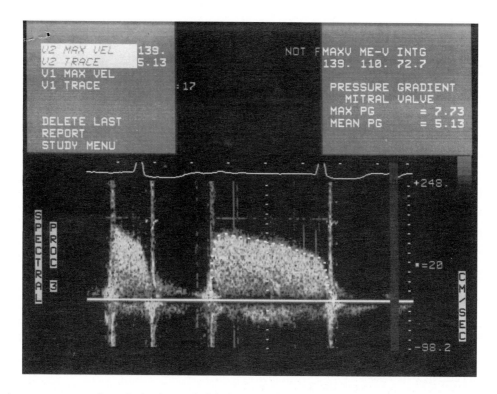

Figure 11.9 Continuous wave recording of mitral stenotic flow in which the flow profile has been planimetered using an on-line Doppler analysis system. This facilitates calculation of the mean mitral valve gradient, which is extremely tedious by manual methods.

as the time taken (in milliseconds) for the peak early diastolic pressure gradient to decline to 50% of its original value. This parameter is known as the pressure half-time.

The velocity equivalent to half the peak pressure may be calculated by multiplying the peak early diastolic velocity by 0.7 (because of the squared relationship between velocity and pressure). Then the point on the declining velocity profile equal to this calculated velocity is found. The pressure half-time is then the time difference between the peak velocity and the calculated point (expressed in milliseconds). The principles of measuring the pressure half-time are illustrated diagrammatically in Figure 11.8.

An empirical formula to calculate the mitral valve area from the half-time was developed by Hatle, so that:

$$\text{Mitral valve area (cm}^2) = \frac{220}{\text{Pressure half-time (ms)}}$$

The velocity decay profile through a stenotic mitral valve is theoretically an exponential. In many patients, especially with mild stenosis, the exponential curve is quite pronounced. However, on many occasions it is clearly a linear decay and a simplification of the above calculation may be performed. To do this, a straight line is drawn on the decay velocity profile so that it is extrapolated to the base line. The time period between the peak velocity and the intercept of the above line with the base line is measured and taken as the "base time". (If the recording paper speed is 1000 mm/s then it is simple to read off these time intervals using a metric ruler.) A geometric simplification of the pressure half-time method results in:

$$\text{Mitral valve area (cm}^2) = \frac{759}{\text{Base time (ms)}}$$

While it is not possible to use this simplified method when the mitral velocity decay profile is curved (since a straight line cannot be drawn down a curve!), it does make calculation of Doppler mitral valve area easier to perform. Above all, it should be remembered that these are empirical formulas that provide an estimate rather than an absolute value for mitral valve area.

Pulmonary and tricuspid stenosis

The Bernouilli equation, as described previously, may be used for calculation of pressure gradients across the right heart valves. Care must again be taken to ensure that the Doppler beam is aligned with the flow profile. This is less of a problem with the pulmonary valve since the main pulmonary artery provides a guide as to the likely jet direction. A mid-precordial transducer position is likely to provide the best beam alignment in tricuspid stenosis. Examples of continuous wave Doppler recordings in pulmonary and tricuspid stenosis are seen in Figures 11.10 and 11.11.

The continuity or pressure half-time methods for valve area estimation have not been validated for the right heart and they should not be used.

Prosthetic valve stenosis

Prosthetic valves may be evaluated in the same way as for native valves except that effective prosthetic orifice area should not be calculated from Doppler since no methods have been reliably validated.

It is possible to use the pressure half-time as a direct parameter to serially follow mitral prostheses. Unfortunately, the normal range of pressure half-times and also pressure gradients for both mitral and aortic prostheses varies considerably depending upon the type, model and size of the prosthesis. It is therefore impossible to quote the normal ranges in this text. However, there have been several large studies performed on most types of valves and the normal data is easily available in the medical literature.

Most prosthetic valves, whether aortic or mitral, are mildly stenotic and therefore one would expect slightly increased peak transvalve velocities. If a baseline postoperative Doppler recording is made following implant, then this probably provides the best reference for further comparison if valve obstruction is suggested at a later date.

Valvular regurgitation

As previously discussed, continuous wave Doppler is more sensitive than pulsed wave. It may therefore be used initially for detecting regurgitant jets, particularly small weak ones.

Pulsed Doppler is used primarily to map the spatial extent of regurgitant jets. It is frequently necessary to map right across the valve in several planes using a variety of views.

The apex is the most commonly used site for continuous wave examination. Since this technique is usually performed "blind" (without imaging), it is theoretically possible to confuse Doppler signals from the following lesions, which may or may not occur in combination: mitral regurgitation, tricuspid regurgitation and aortic stenosis, and aortic regurgitation and mitral stenosis.

Figure 11.12 illustrates diagrammatically the possible combination of flow signals that may occur in mixed left heart valve disease. To ensure that we know exactly what signals are being recorded the following pointers should be used:

1. Confirmation of site of abnormal jets using pulsed Doppler.
2. Duration, shape, timing and position of abnormal jet.
3. Peak velocity and position of peak.
4. Shape of forward flow profile, no reverse flow interval.

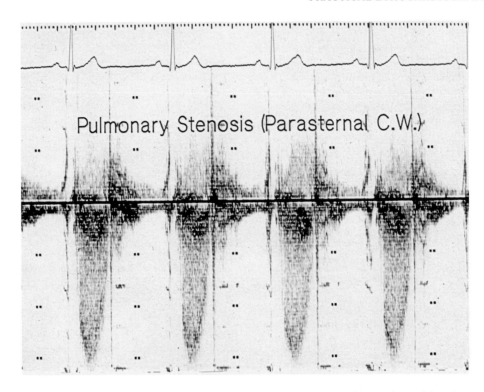

Figure 11.10 Continuous wave Doppler recording of flow through the pulmonary valve in a patient with pulmonary stenosis. Systolic flow of approximately 3 m/s is seen going away from the transducer. The peak pulmonary valve gradient is therefore calculated at 35 mmHg.

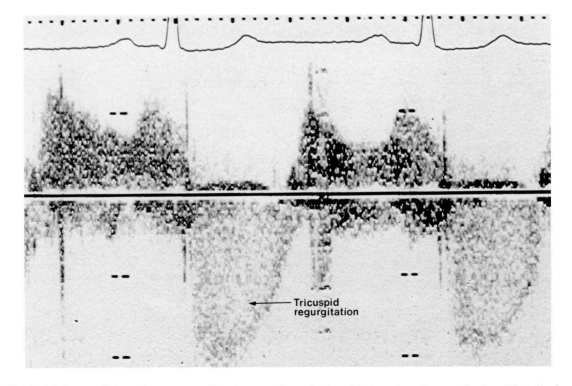

Figure 11.11 Mid-precordial continuous wave Doppler recording of tricuspid stenosis and regurgitation. Diastolic flow through the tricuspid valve is slightly increased in peak velocity (1.3 m/s) and has a reduced rate of descent. In systole, flow away from the transducer arising from tricuspid regurgitation is seen. This flow velocity is 2 m/s and does not suggest the presence of pulmonary hypertension since the right ventricular systolic pressure is calculated at 16 mmHg plus the jugular venous pressure.

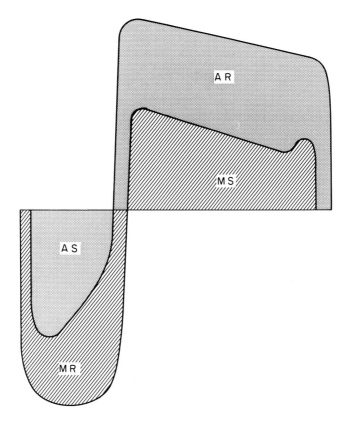

Figure 11.12 Diagrammatic representation of the possible continuous wave flow profiles that may be recorded in patients with multiple left-sided valvular lesions. It is important to note that all flow signals arising from the same valve are continuous with one another, so that there is no time delay when forward flow through the aortic valve in systole becomes retrograde regurgitant flow during diastole. This latter point is helpful in identifying the origin of flow signals. In addition, it is normal to find that the velocity, shape and duration of flow signals will vary depending upon the valvular lesion responsible. For example, aortic regurgitation should always be higher in velocity and longer in duration than flow through the mitral valve (whether stenotic or not). Both of these flow patterns would be moving toward the transducer (positioned at the apex) in diastole. For further explanation see text.

The use of the above pointers will become more apparent in the following specific sections. It is important to remember that the peak velocity of a regurgitant jet does *not* correlate with severity. It is merely a reflection of the pressure difference across the valve; however this fact can help in separating flows from different valvular lesions, for example mitral versus tricuspid regurgitation or aortic regurgitation versus mitral stenosis.

Aortic regurgitation

This hemodynamic lesion is best detected using an apical transducer position and by looking for diastolic high velocity flow in the left ventricular outflow tract. Small jets from very mild lesions can require considerable searching across the valve with the pulsed Doppler sample volume. Pulsed Doppler recordings will almost certainly be aliased, whereas continuous wave will demonstrate flow toward the transducer which should be well above 3 m/s in early diastole (unlike mitral stenosis). Forward and reversed flows across the same valve will be continuous with one another. This means that, as the regurgitant signal stops, the forward aortic flow should be immediately visible with no time interval between them. This factor is very helpful in confirming the site of flow signal.

Some idea of severity can be achieved by mapping the length and width of the regurgitant jet (within the left ventricle) using pulsed Doppler. This is based upon the premise that more significant and larger volume regurgitant jets will extend further into the ventricle. Examples of pulsed Doppler recordings both in the left ventricular outflow tract and mapping back into the left ventricle are seen in Figures 11.13 and 11.14.

Unfortunately, the length and width of regurgitant jets are dependent not only on the regurgitant volume but also on the driving pressure and hence the velocity of the jet.

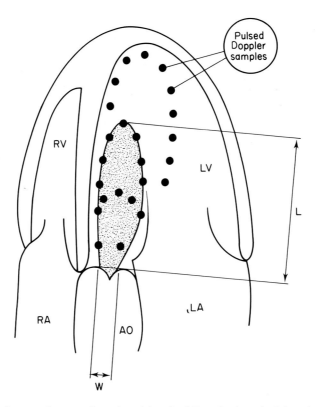

Figure 11.13 Systematic mapping of an aortic regurgitant jet with pulsed Doppler in apical five chamber view. The shaded area shows how, when the spatial extent of the jet has been identified, its length and width may be calculated. The apical five chamber view is obtained by angling the transducer scan plane anteriorly from the four chamber view (Figure 2.3e). This brings the left ventricular outflow tract, aortic valve and aortic root into the scan plane. This view is probably inappropriately named since the aorta is not a chamber.

This does limit the use of this single criterion for quantitative analysis of all regurgitant lesions. However, severity can usually be separated into mild, moderate or severe categories on the basis that mild regurgitant jets are usually limited to the outflow tract, moderate jets may extend midway down the ventricle (to the mitral leaflet tips) and severe jets will usually penetrate to the apex. The length and width of all regurgitant jets should be mapped out in at least two orthogonal because since they are themselves three-dimensional. Since we are not trying to measure velocity but to establish the spatial existence of a flow disturbance, it is not essential to be aligned parallel to flow and parasternal views may be used for pulsed Doppler jet mapping. In patients with coexistent mitral stenosis it may be difficult to map the aortic regurgitant jet if it mixes with high velocity flow through the mitral valve.

On continuous wave Doppler, mitral diastolic flow may be separated from aortic regurgitation because the latter will always be higher in velocity (<3 m/s in early diastole), if the patient is in sinus rythmn then the mitral profile will have a biphasic shape (from early and late diastolic filling), and finally aortic regurgitant flow will be continuous with forward flow through the aortic valve. An example of

aortic regurgitation on continuous wave Doppler is seen in Figure 11.15.

If the continuous wave recording is of good spectral quality, some appreciation of regurgitation severity may be achieved by comparing the intensity of the forward and reversed flows through the valve. The spectral intensity is dependent on the number of red blood cells within the Doppler beam, and if the forward and reversed flow intensities are similar, then the regurgitation is usually at least moderate in severity.

In patients with significant aortic regurgitant flow, the aortic diastolic pressure will be reduced (with a wide pulse pressure) and hence the aorta to left ventricle end-diastolic gradient and velocity will be low. The rate of descent of the diastolic portion of the flow profile is therefore proportional to the severity of regurgitation. In patients with trivial aortic regurgitation, the beginning and end-diastolic jet velocities will be similar, whereas in severe regurgitation the end-diastolic velocity is much lower. The rate of descent can be measured in terms of velocity half-time. In severe regurgitation half-time is approximately 0.5 s and in moderate regurgitation it is approximately 1 s. This parameter is dependent upon other factors such as aortic and left

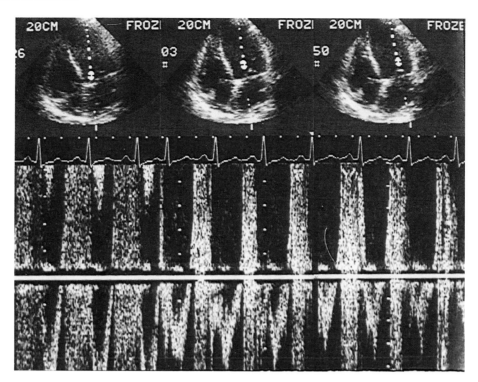

Figure 11.14 Pulsed Doppler mapping of aortic regurgitation using an apical five chamber view. Three of the many pulse Doppler sampler positions are shown and in this example the flow jet is tracked from the left ventricular outflow tract across to the mitral valve orifice. As diagrammatically illustrated in Figure 11.13, multiple sample volume positions are utilized throughout the left ventricle using as many imaging planes as possible.

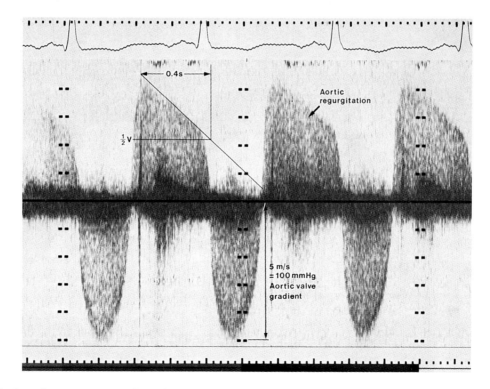

Figure 11.15 Apical continuous wave recording of aortic stenosis and regurgitation. The peak aortic pressure gradient is calculated at approximately 100 mmHg. On the basis of this recording, the regurgitation would be graded as severe in that the regurgitant jet has significant intensity and a rapid rate of spectral diastolic descent with a regurgitant half-time of less than 0.5 s.

ventricular compliance, mitral filling and left ventricular diastolic pressure. However, with these limitations in mind, a short velocity half-time is, in practice, a reliable indicator of severe regurgitation.

It is theoretically possible to calculate the left ventricular end-diastolic pressure (and in the absence of mitral stenosis, the left atrial pressure) by subtracting the end-diastolic aorta to left ventricle pressure gradient from a cuff diastolic blood pressure reading. The pressure gradient is calculated in the usual manner using $4V^2$ and the end-diastolic regurgitant velocity. Unfortunately, it can be difficult to satisfactorily record diastolic blood pressure in patients with significant aortic regurgitation and this limits the usefulness of the technique.

In patients with severe aortic regurgitation, retrograde diastolic flow may be detectable (using either pulsed or continuous wave Doppler) in the ascending or descending aorta and occasionally the carotid and subclavian arteries. Initial reversal of flow in early diastole is normal (Figure 11.16), but if the reversed flow is continuous throughout diastole then the regurgitation is significant. An example of retrograde diastolic flow in the descending aorta is seen in Figure 11.17.

Mitral regurgitation

This lesion is usually best detected from the apex, using either pulsed or continuous wave Doppler. With the transducer in this position, most regurgitant jets will be directed away in a superior direction. However, if the jet is directed posteriorly, then a parasternal transducer position may be better.

Unless there is a need to accurately record the flow profile and peak velocity, it is obviously not vital to be lined up with the jet. Systolic turbulence within the left atrium can be picked up on pulsed or continuous wave Doppler even if the Doppler beam is perpendicular to the jet direction. Therefore, as previously mentioned, detecting and mapping the spatial extent of mitral regurgitant jets can be performed using either parasternal or apical windows, preferably both. Mild lesions demonstrate systolic turbulence only immediately behind the leaflets, whereas severe mitral regurgitant jets will be detectable at the most superior aspect of the left atrium and will be reasonably broad. An example of severe mitral regurgitation mapped to the superior aspect of the left atrium is seen in Figure 11.18. In patients with mitral valve prolapse, the jets are often very eccentric and

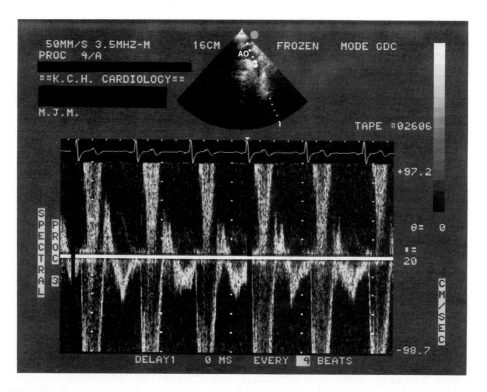

Figure 11.16 Pulsed Doppler recording with two sample volumes positioned in the proximal portion of the descending aorta and the transducer in a suprasternal position. Systolic flow down the descending aorta is away from the transducer. However, in this recording the signal is aliased (3.5 MHz transducer used). In diastole an initial reversal of flow toward the transducer is seen and then, throughout the remainder of diastole, low velocity flow continues down the descending aorta.

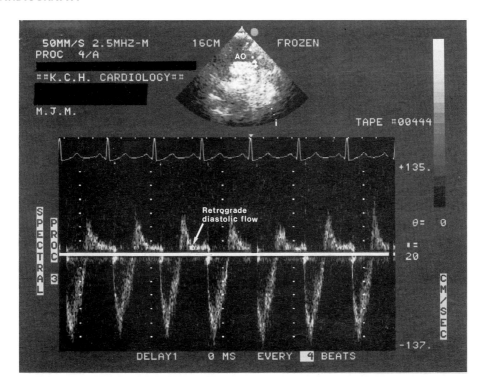

Figure 11.17 In this patient with severe aortic regurgitation, diastolic retrograde flow toward the transducer (in the descending aorta) continues throughout diastole. Laminar flow during systole is seen traveling away from the transducer.

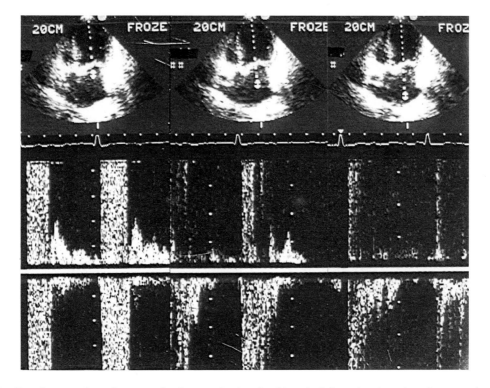

Figure 11.18 Pulse Doppler mapping of severe mitral regurgitation. In this apical four chamber view the regurgitant jet is mapped to the most superior aspect of the left atrium and was also found to be broad.

will usually be directed behind the leaflet that is prolapsing least, as shown in Figure 11.19.

On continuous wave Doppler recordings, it is important to check that the mitral regurgitant jet is continuous with the typical mitral forward flow pattern to exclude the possibility of recording aortic stenotic flow, the latter usually having a more peaked profile. If the velocity is under 3–4 m/s then the recording may be of tricuspid regurgitation. This has a longer duration than mitral regurgitation and is recorded with a more medial transducer angulation.

As with aortic regurgitant jets on continuous wave Doppler, the intensity of the forward and reversed flow signals should be compared to obtain some idea of severity. Mild mitral regurgitant jets are not usually recorded throughout systole because the jets are narrow and may move in and out of the Doppler beam as the mitral annulus changes orientation during systole.

In patients with severe mitral regurgitation, the left atrial pressure rises significantly during systole, causing the char-

acteristic "v" waves seen at cardiac catheterization. This phenomenon is evident on continuous wave recordings as an early systolic fall in the jet velocity as the ventricle-to-atrium pressure gradient drops. Mitral regurgitant jets normally have a rounded systolic profile as seen in Figure 11.20. However when "v" waves are present the peak velocity is in early systole; this is illustrated in Figure 11.21.

Pulmonary regurgitation

Mild pulmonary regurgitation is a common finding, especially in children and patients with pulmonary hypertension. It is possible to confuse normal tricuspid flow with tricuspid regurgitation. In addition, when using continuous wave Doppler, other signals from mitral valve or coronary artery flow may be mistaken for pulmonary regurgitation.

An example of pulmonary regurgitation recorded using pulsed Doppler is seen in Figure 11.22. The degree of regurgitation is assessed using the signal intensity (on continuous wave)' and jet extension into the right ventricle as mapped by pulsed Doppler. The rate of decrease of the regurgitant velocity signal may be used qualitatively to establish severity. However, there have been no quantitative studies reported, as with aortic regurgitation, presumably because of the lack of a suitable gold standard with which to assess pulmonary regurgitation.

Pulmonary artery diastolic pressure can be estimated by using the end-diastolic pulmonary regurgitant jet velocity to calculate the pressure difference between the pulmonary artery and the right ventricle (modified Bernouilli equation). The right ventricular diastolic pressure should equal the right atrial and jugular venous pressure in the absence of tricuspid stenosis. Hence the pulmonary artery diastolic pressure equals the right ventricle to pulmonary artery pressure difference plus the jugular venous pressure. The latter can be measured using conventional noninvasive techniques or simply taken as approximately 5 mmHg.

Tricuspid regurgitation

Tricuspid regurgitation is also surprisingly common in normal people, with several studies reporting incidences of well over 40%. In patients with significant cardiac pathology, tricuspid regurgitation is almost invariably found. Since the tricuspid valve is such a complex structure, it is probably not surprising that mild or trivial regurgitation is so common. In fact, recent studies using transesophageal echo Doppler have established that trivial regurgitation is a physiological feature of most normal valves, especially as they close at the beginning of systole.

The direction of tricuspid jets is very variable and it is often necessary to search carefully with both pulsed and continuous wave Doppler using parasternal, apical and subcostal views.

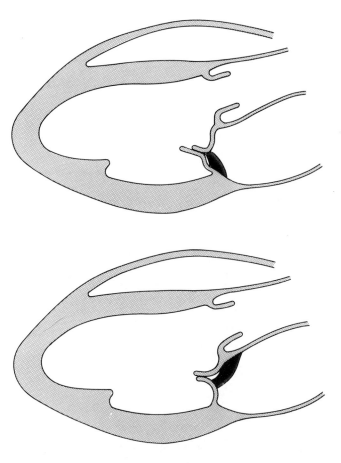

Figure 11.19a Diagram showing how, in patients with mitral valve prolapse, the regurgitant jet is usually directed behind the leaflet which is prolapsing least. This provides a useful indicator when searching for the small eccentric jets that can occur in this condition.

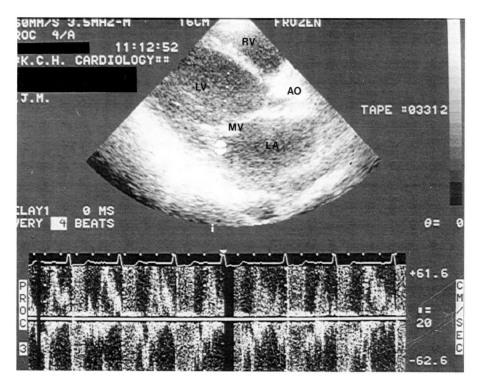

Figure 11.19b In this patient, in whom the mitral valve prolapse mainly involves the anterior leaflet, the regurgitant jet is detected with the sample volume positioned behind the posterior leaflet. In systole, a high velocity aliased signal from mitral regurgitation is seen on the pulsed Doppler recording.

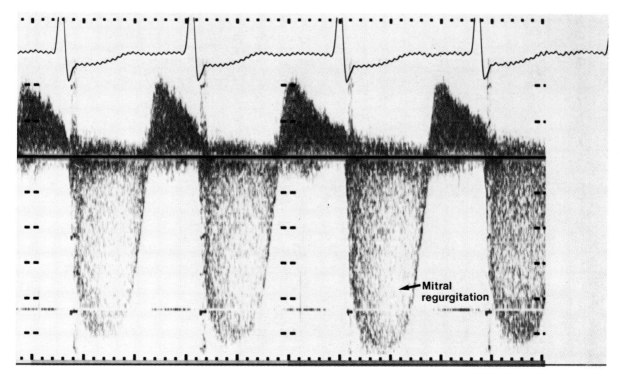

Figure 11.20 Apical continuous wave Doppler recording of mild to moderate mitral regurgitation. The mitral regurgitant jet has a fairly low spectral intensity, particularly in mid-systole, and has the classic rounded shape with peak velocity occurring in mid-systole.

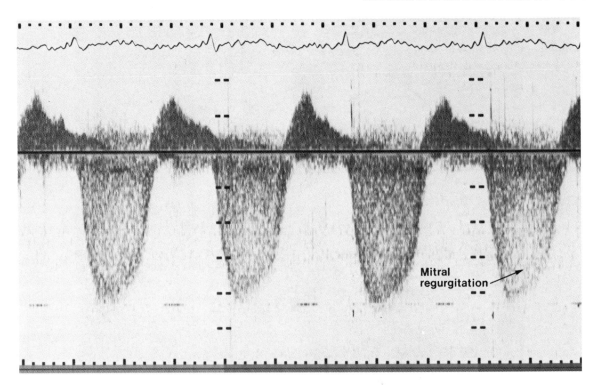

Mitral regurgitation

Figure 11.21   In this patient with more severe mitral regurgitation and left atrial "v" waves, the peak jet velocity occurs in early systole. As the left atrial pressure rises during systole, the left atrial-to-ventricular pressure gradient reduces and consequently the regurgitant jet velocity decreases.

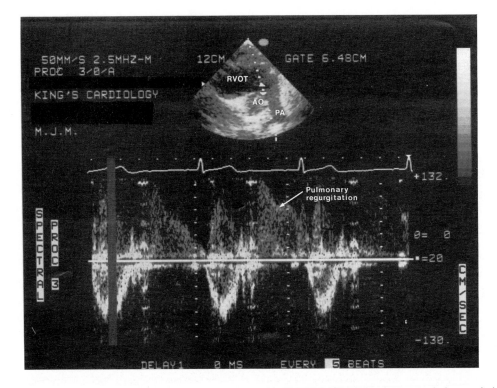

Figure 11.22   Pulsed Doppler recording from the right ventricular outflow tract utilizing the parasternal short axis imaging plane in a patient with mild pulmonary regurgitation. In systole the flow is directed away from the transducer toward the pulmonary valve, and in diastole regurgitant flow toward the transducer is seen.

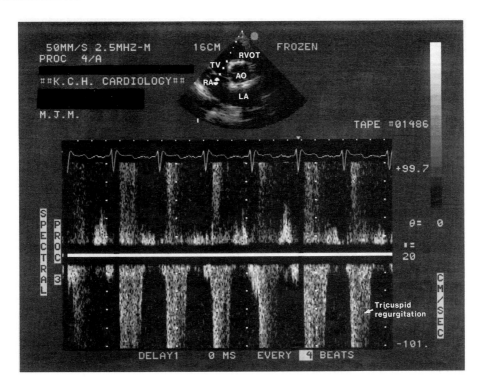

Figure 11.23 Pulsed Doppler recording of tricuspid regurgitation from a parasternal short axis view. Tricuspid regurgitant jets are often very eccentric and should be mapped using multiple imaging planes so that the true spatial extent may be appreciated. In this view, abnormal systolic flow is seen behind the tricuspid valve which has a high velocity and is aliased.

Severity of regurgitation is judged by the usual methods of mapping the spatial extent of the jet, as shown in Figure 11.23. Mild regurgitation will be evident just behind the valve leaflets, moderate jets will extend to the superior atrial wall, and in severe regurgitation turbulent retrograde flow will be detected in the hepatic veins (using subcostal views). It is also important to examine the signal intensity on continuous wave. An example of tricuspid regurgitation on continuous wave Doppler is shown in Figure 11.24. The jet is usually longer in duration, lower in velocity and found with a more medial transducer angulation than mitral regurgitation. In patients with right ventricular failure, the rate of jet velocity increase is often reduced.

Pulmonary artery systolic pressure can be very reliably estimated using the peak systolic velocity of the tricuspid regurgitant jet. The right atrial to right ventricular systolic pressure difference can be calculated using the Bernouilli formula ($4V^2$) and the peak jet velocity. This pressure difference is then added to the right atrial or jugular venous pressure (measured by conventional methods or taken as 5 mmHg) to give the ventricular systolic pressure. In the absence of pulmonary valve stenosis, this will equal the pulmonary artery systolic pressure. The principle of calculating pulmonary artery systolic pressure from the tricuspid regurgitant jet velocity is shown diagrammatically in Figure 11.25. In patients with cardiac pathology (especially pulmonary hypertension), tricuspid regurgitation is so common that it is possible to estimate the pulmonary artery pressure in most cases. This has been shown in several studies to be very accurate and, of course, is clinically extremely useful. In Figure 11.24 the peak jet velocity is 4 m/s giving a pulmonary artery systolic pressure of $4 \times 4^2 +$ jugular venous pressure, i.e. approximately 70 mmHg.

Prosthetic valve regurgitation

Prosthetic valves are assessed very much as for native valves. However, since jets are often very eccentric and in addition the prosthesis may cause masking of the regurgitant Doppler signal, unconventional views may be required.

Simultaneous imaging and Doppler is needed to distinguish between valvular and paravalvar leaks. It may be impossible to make this distinction in many cases, particularly with an aortic prosthesis because the left ventricular outflow tract is relatively small and it is difficult to just sample around the sewing ring of the valve.

It is frequently helpful to use parasternal short axis views of the left ventricular outflow tract and left atrium when evaluating regurgitation in aortic and mitral prostheses respectively. In these views, the prosthesis should not mask

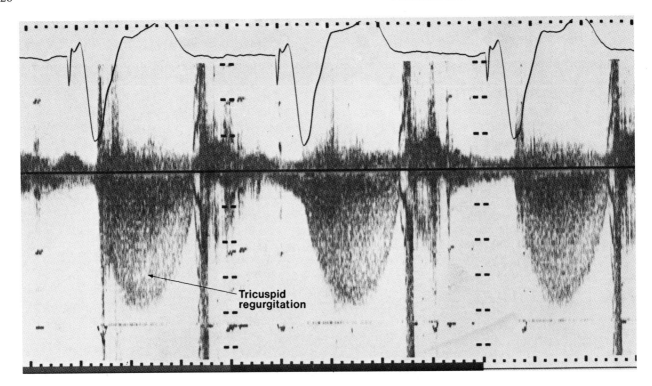

Figure 11.24 Continuous wave recording of tricuspid regurgitation in a patient with a pacemaker. The tricuspid regurgitant jet is relatively long in duration and, because this patient has pulmonary hypertension, the peak velocity is increased at approximately 4 m/s (see text for explanation).

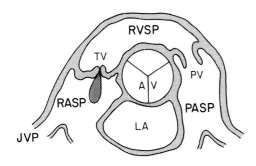

Figure 11.25 Diagram illustrating how, by measuring tricuspid regurgitant jet velocity, it is possible (in patients without pulmonary stenosis) to calculate the systolic pressure difference between the pulmonary artery and right atrium.

$$PASP = RVSP$$
$$RVSP = RASP + 4V^2$$
$$RASP = JVP$$
$$\therefore \ PASP = JVP + 4V^2$$

the regurgitant jet and the spatial position of any turbulent flow can be detected. An example of the use of this technique in a patient with a paravalvar aortic leak is seen in Figure 11.26.

The increased sensitivity of continuous wave Doppler does mean that regurgitant jets are more regularly detected with this technique. However, valvular and paravalvar leaks are usually indistinguishable from one another. In addition, it is apparent that most metal prostheses are naturally slightly regurgitant and these normal, trivial jets are frequently seen on continuous wave Doppler examination and color flow mapping.

The severity of prosthetic valve regurgitation may be evaluated using conventional methods such as the relative intensity of the continuous wave Doppler signal and the extension of the jet into the receiving chamber. However, since prosthetic jets are often very eccentric, it may be difficult to use the latter technique reliably.

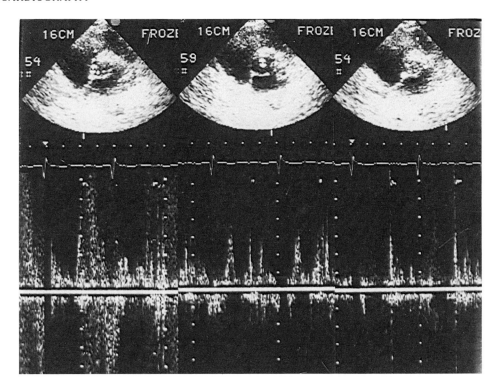

Figure 11.26 Pulsed Doppler mapping across the left ventricular outflow tract using the short axis imaging plane in a patient with paraprosthetic aortic regurgitation. As shown in the left-hand recording, a diastolic flow disturbance is detected on the medial aspect of the outflow tract. However, as the sample volume is moved across to the central and lateral aspect of the outflow tract no flow disturbance is detected. This examination suggested a medial paraprosthetic leak which was indeed confirmed by angiography.

Congenital heart disease

Congenital valvular lesions such as a bicuspid aortic valve can be hemodynamically assessed in the same way as described for acquired valve disease. Subvalvar and infundibular stenotic gradients can also be measured by applying the peak recorded velocity to the modified Bernouilli equation as described before. However, dynamic infundibular obstruction produces a characteristic (continuous wave) Doppler signal with a gradually accelerating systolic velocity as shown in Figure 11.27. This allows easy identification of both the infundibular and valvular components of serial stenotic lesions which may occur, for example, in pulmonary stenosis.

Pulsed Doppler can play a very useful role in documenting the site of intracardiac shunts. Small atrial or ventricular septal defects are often not easily seen on standard echo imaging. However, because they are small, the flow velocity across these defects is usually high and easy to recognize during the Doppler examination. Using as many views as possible, the pulsed Doppler sample volume is moved along the septal surface (usually on the right heart side) until an abnormal flow pattern is detected. In Figure 11.28 the sample volume has been placed directly adjacent to a small perimembranous outflow ventricular septal defect. A high velocity jet coming from the right to the left ventricle is seen. With larger defects, the volume of blood flow will be higher and more significant but the velocity lower. This may make Doppler detection more difficult; however large defects are usually easy to directly visualize on 2D echo. Since continuous wave Doppler is more sensitive than pulsed Doppler, it is often easier to detect ventricular septal defect jets using this technique. If the continuous wave transducer is moved over the left parasternal edge and precordium, and a high velocity systolic jet toward the transducer is recorded (as shown in Figure 11.29), then this must be considered strongly suggestive of ventricular septal defect flow. If a high quality and well-defined signal is recorded, then it is possible to use the Bernouilli equation to calculate the systolic pressure difference between the two ventricles. The absolute right ventricular and pulmonary artery systolic pressure can then be measured by subtracting this pressure from the systemic systolic pressure (obtained by arm cuff).

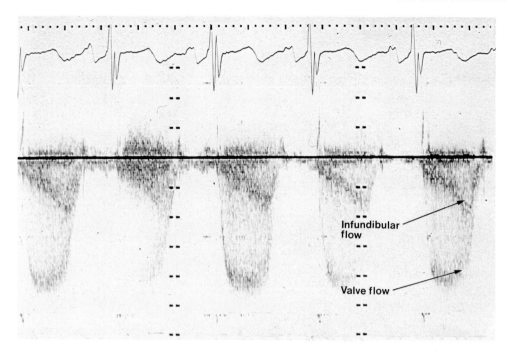

Figure 11.27 Parasternal continuous wave recording through the right ventricular outflow tract and pulmonary valve in a patient with infundibular and valvular pulmonary stenosis. The infundibular stenosis is mild and may be recognized by the gradually accelerating systolic flow profile with a peak velocity of 2 m/s. The valvular component is severe, the velocity profile rising rapidly here to a peak of 4 m/s.

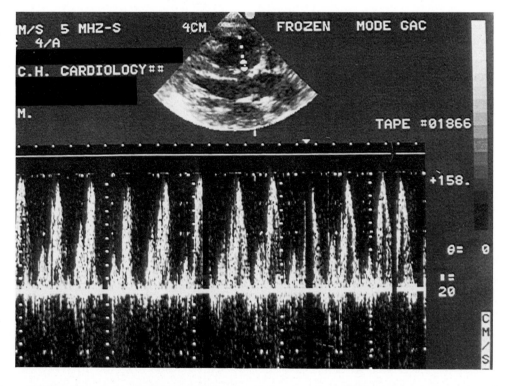

Figure 11.28 The pulsed Doppler sample volume is placed directly adjacent to an area of echo dropout in the perimembranous ventricular septum. The flow is seen coming toward the transducer into the right ventricle, confirming that this is indeed a ventricular septal defect. It is important to establish that suspected ventricular septal defect flow jets are not indeed arising from the tricuspid valve and this may be done by using the ECG (for timing purposes) if available.

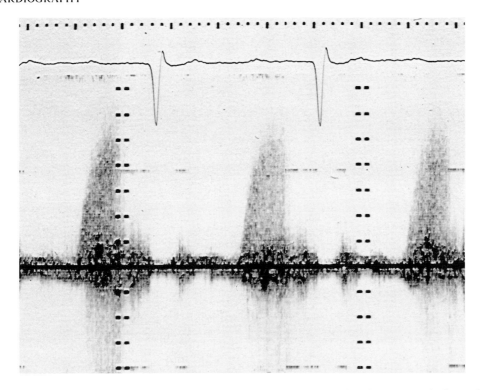

Figure 11.29 Ventricular septal defect jet recorded using continuous wave Doppler on the left parasternal edge. A high velocity systolic flow is seen traveling toward the transducer. The peak velocity is over 5 m/s, suggesting a high pressure differential between the left and right ventricles and virtually excluding the presence of significant pulmonary hypertension.

Patent ductus arteriosus can be very difficult to image, especially in the neonate. The flow of blood into the pulmonary artery from the aorta results in abnormal retrograde diastolic and occasionally continuous pulmonary flow. This is very easy to detect using pulsed and continuous wave Doppler and has made the technique both highly sensitive and specific for the diagnosis of patent ductus. An example of retrograde pulmonary artery flow in this condition is seen in Figure 11.30.

Coarctation of the aorta is another congenital pathology that has characteristic Doppler findings. Coarctation nearly always occurs in the descending aorta just distal to the left subclavian artery. The obstruction causes an increase in systolic blood velocity with prolonged forward flow during diastole in the descending aorta (especially in patients with extensive collaterals). This can be easily detected with a continuous wave transducer placed in the suprasternal position. An example is illustrated in Figure 11.31. By altering the angulation of the transducer it is possible to record ascending and descending aortic flow velocities. The increase in descending aortic velocity is related to the degree of obstruction. The pressure gradient across the obstruction can be calculated as previously described for stenotic valves. In patients who also have patent ductus, the ductal flow will

tend to reduce the pressure gradient and Doppler diagnosis is less reliable.

Color flow mapping is invaluable for detecting and evaluating the very complex flow patterns that may occur in congenital heart disease. This is discussed briefly later in this chapter.

Flow calculations

It is important to remember that Doppler measures blood velocity and not volumetric flow rate. However, systemic and/or pulmonary flow volumes can be calculated from the blood velocities in the aorta and pulmonary artery respectively. If one assumes that the aorta and pulmonary artery are cylinders (their cross-sectional areas can be measured by standard echo techniques), then the volume of blood flow with each cardiac cycle is the area multiplied by the stroke distance. This in effect calculates the stroke volume and in the absence of any intracardiac shunt should be the same for both the right and left heart. If the stroke volume is multiplied by the heart rate then the cardiac output is calculated.

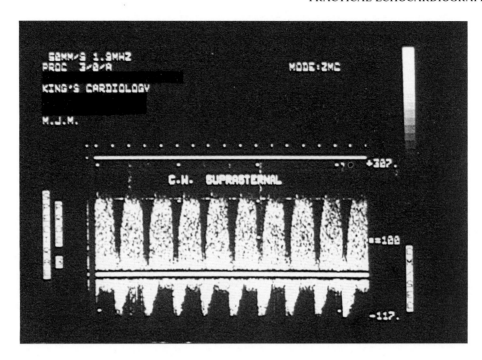

Figure 11.30   Suprasternal continuous wave Doppler recording in a patient with patent ductus arteriosus. Systolic flow away from the transducer down the pulmonary artery is seen and the high velocity jet arising from flow through the duct is detected traveling toward the transducer in diastole.

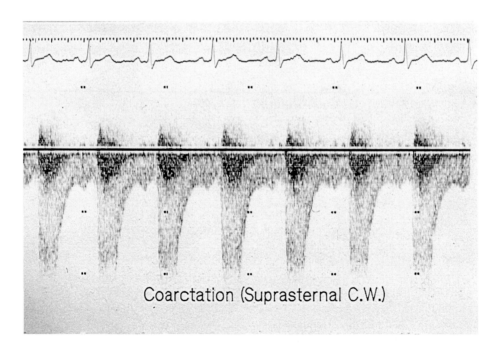

Figure 11.31   The classical suprasternal continuous wave recording from coarctation of the aorta is seen here. The peak systolic profile is not well defined and therefore it would be inappropriate to estimate the coarctation gradient from this recording. However, continuous low velocity flow through the coarctation (and any collaterals) is seen during diastole.

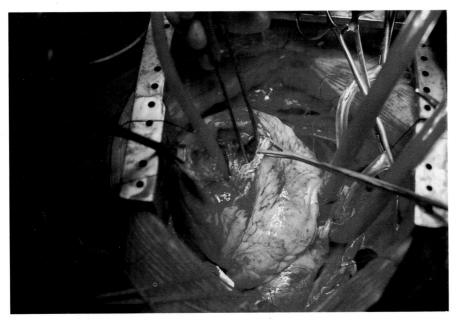

Plate 7.1
Intraoperative photograph of the repair of a postinfarct ventricular septal defect. The apex of the heart has been opened and deflected upwards so that the interventricular septum can be seen running across the center (next to the cannula entering the left ventricle). The defect is therefore positioned in the apical portion of the interventricular septum, as predicted by the echocardiogram of the patient, which is shown in Figure 7.6.

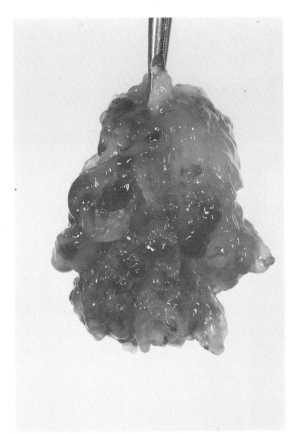

Plate 9.1
A typical left atrial myxoma. It is suspended by the forceps from the narrow stalk which attaches the tumor to the interatrial septum. The structure is large and jelly-like, and has a slightly narrowed, waisted portion where the mitral valve leaflets wrapped around it during diastole.

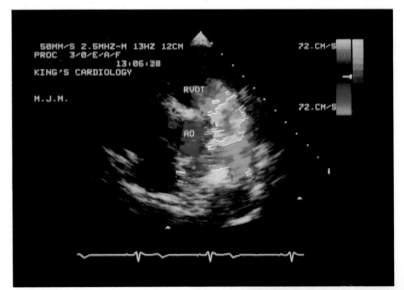

Plate 11.1
Parasternal short axis view of systolic flow in the main pulmonary artery visualized using color flow mapping. Flow down the pulmonary artery is away from the transducer and color encoded as blue. However, at the origin of the pulmonary artery the flow velocity exceeds the Nyquist limit and aliases through to yellow and red.

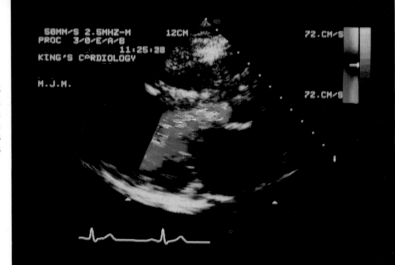

Plate 11.2
Color flow image of aortic regurgitation using a parasternal long axis view. The main component of flow is away from the transducer and therefore encoded as blue although there is some aliasing through to red. Variance mapping has been employed in this example and consequently green is also seen within the flow jet since it is turbulent.

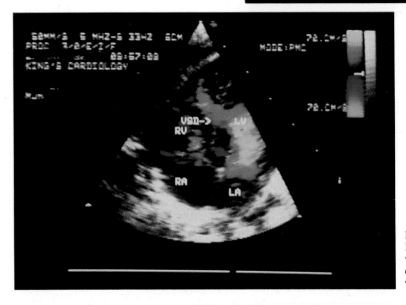

Plate 11.3
Modified four chamber view in a patient with a muscular ventricular septal defect. Flow through the defect is encoded red as it moves toward the transducer into the right ventricle.

Plate 11.4

In this apical four chamber color flow image severe mitral and tricuspid regurgitation can be seen. This patient also has a secundum atrial septal defect and the regurgitant jets from both the atrioventricular valves appear to cross over through the defect. This type of complex flow pattern would be impossible to evaluate using conventional pulsed Doppler mapping.

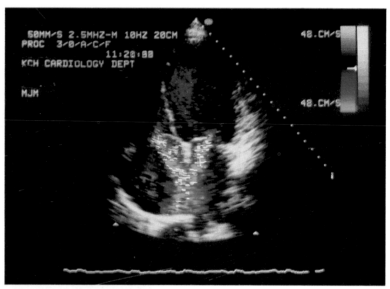

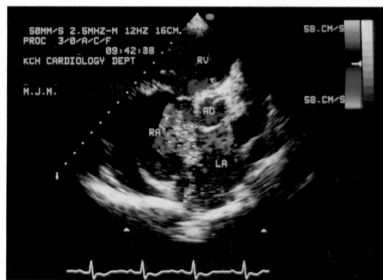

Plate 11.5

Color flow image of left-to-right shunting through a secundum atrial septal defect. Flow is seen entering the left atrium through the pulmonary veins and then crossing the defect where it aliases slightly to blue as it enters the right atrium.

The stroke distance is calculated by measuring the area under the systolic flow profile and is equivalent to the distance moved by the red blood cells with each systole. Thus there are two major components to the calculation of volumetric blood flow: measurement of the vessel cross-sectional area and measurement of the stroke distance from the Doppler systolic flow profile. Ideally, of course, these measurements should occur at the same point in the vessel.

Velocity measurements should not be made in sites where nonlaminar flow exists. For example, ascending aortic flow will be turbulent in patients with aortic stenosis, subaortic obstruction and prosthetic valves. Wherever possible, attempts should be made to align the Doppler beam parallel with flow and record the highest velocity, preferably near the origin of the aorta or pulmonary artery where the spatial velocity profile will be relatively flat.

As mentioned previously, the stroke distance is the area under the systolic flow profile and is best and most conveniently calculated using either a semiautomatic on-line or off-line Doppler analysis system. The modal flow velocity is traced into the computer, which automatically calculates the stroke distance for each beat. The modal rather than the peak or mean velocity is chosen for analysis because this represents that velocity at which most red blood cells are traveling (the darkest part of the spectral flow curve). In addition, several studies have shown that the best correlation with other techniques is achieved when the modal velocity is used. Since there can be some beat-to-beat variation in the stroke distance, an average of five or six cardiac cycles should be used. This is another good reason for using a computerized analysis system since manual planimetry methods can be extremely tedious.

The vessel cross-sectional area may be calculated by measuring the diameter (in systole) and using the formula

$$\text{Area} = \pi(\text{diameter}/2)^2$$

This of course assumes that the vessel is circular in cross-section and that the true diameter is being measured. (Care must be taken to achieve this since any errors are squared.) When measuring the pulmonary artery diameter, this has to be done using the lateral resolution of 2D imaging and may introduce further errors, particularly if the lateral pulmonary artery wall is poorly visualized, as is frequently the case. It is of course possible to directly visualize the aortic root in cross-section and the area could be directly planimetered. However, errors may again be introduced by poor lateral resolution and any obliquity of the scan plane. Measurement of vessel cross-sectional area is undoubtedly the largest source of error in this technique. For this reason, many centers prefer to utilize stroke distance alone for serial comparisons within the same patient.

There have been many proposed sites and methods for Doppler measurement of cardiac output. However, best results have been achieved if the velocity and diameter are measured at the site of the aortic orifice. In this position, the site for Doppler and velocity measurement is sharply defined and reproducible, the smallest aortic diameter is measured, and a flat spatial velocity profile is most likely at this level.

Using parasternal views, the diameter and cross-sectional area of the aortic orifice can be measured (in systole, as shown in Figure 11.32). Then utilizing apical windows, the pulsed Doppler sample volume can be positioned in precisely the same anatomical position to allow the flow velocity measurements to be made with the Doppler beam aligned parallel to flow.

While the aorta is most commonly used for cardiac output measurements, it is also frequently possible to measure it using the pulmonary artery. Some studies have, in addition, suggested mitral and tricuspid flow as further alternative sites for measurement. However, there are significant practical difficulties in utilizing these sites, and they are not widely used.

In theory, by analyzing flow in the aorta and pulmonary artery, this technique will not only measure the cardiac output but also allow comparison of systemic and pulmonary flows and therefore shunt ratios. In practice there are a number of technical difficulties, including the calculation of mean velocity which requires computer assistance and the measurement of vessel area which is prone to errors. However, in experienced hands this technique has been shown to be reliable and provides a convenient method of calculating the hemodynamic significance of shunts and also cardiac output.

Color flow mapping

Perhaps the most exciting recent Doppler innovation is that of color flow mapping. Superficially, real-time color flow images have the appearance of a colored angiogram, where cardiac blood flow is depicted using a color code to illustrate blood velocity and direction. The color coded blood flow data is superimposed, in real-time, onto the 2D image so that a spatially oriented map of blood flow information is obtained. This may be correlated with anatomical information from the conventional ultrasound image. The blood flow data may also be superimposed onto an M-Mode recording. This may be particularly useful for exact timing of flow in relation to mechanical intracardiac events.

By convention, blood flow away from the transducer is colored blue with an increase in brightness or change in hue for the higher velocities. Flow toward the transducer is displayed as red with higher velocities again shown in increasing brightness or changing hue through to yellow.

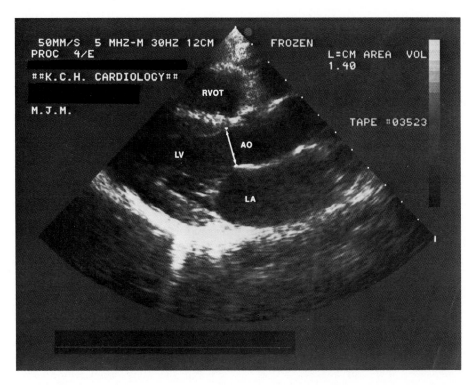

Figure 11.32 Systolic parasternal long axis view showing the point of measurement of the diameter of the aortic orifice. This diameter measurement may then be used to calculate the aortic orifice area. Then using an apical long axis view, the pulsed Doppler sample volume may be placed in precisely the same anatomical location for recording the systolic flow profile and calculating stroke distance.

The exact system of coloration will depend both on the map selected and the instrument used.

The technique uses a modification of pulsed Doppler technology – autocorrelation – to acquire mean blood velocity and direction data down a selected number of image scan lines. The number of data points or sample volumes on each line, and hence the axial resolution of the instrument, can vary from under 100 to over 400 depending on the manufacturer.

Each line of Doppler data must be sampled several consecutive times to obtain both reliable flow and image data. It is impossible to do this for each of the 100 or so lines in an image, perform up to 400 flow calculations per line, and yet still achieve a frame rate which will produce a diagnostic moving image. This is particularly a problem in pediatric cases where the heart rate may be very high. Therefore, some compromise in the number of scan lines used for color flow data is usually necessary. To achieve this, the width or sector angle of the color image may be reduced to 30° or 45° and flow data collected on only alternate scan lines. This has the unfortunate consequence of reducing the spatial resolution.

Recently available ultra high speed microprocessors have improved the processing speed of the flow calculations so

that frame rates of, for example, 14 Hz at 16 cm over a 45° color flow sector arc are now obtainable. Note that most conventional 2D images are displayed at 30 Hz over a 90° sector arc, more than double the color flow frame rate. Again, some manufacturers have been more successful in achieving acceptable frame rates than others and this is an important parameter for equipment evaluation. Low frame rates are distracting, causing flicker in a real-time image and important information may be missed.

Using conventional Doppler techniques, the presence of turbulent blood flow is inferred by "spectral broadening" in the flow signal. Since color flow mapping is only capable of displaying the mean blood velocity at any point, turbulence may not be detected by the use of spectral broadening. An alternative method using "variance mapping" is therefore employed. In this technique, the spatial and temporal statistical variation in blood flow velocity and direction around every color flow pixel is measured. If there is a high variance in the flow signals, then the blood flow at that point is assumed to be turbulent. The color green is then added, at that point, to the other colors that would have been displayed. Variance or turbulence mapping is an option on most instruments and, when used, areas of turbulent flow are easily recognized by the presence of green color. Theoretically, it is possible to quantitate the amount of variance, and hence turbulence, present in a flow jet. In the future, this may have a number of important applications, including the serial monitoring of valve function.

As with conventional 2D imaging, artefacts in color flow images may arise as a result of poor insonation between the transducer and the heart. Lung and rib interference may cause a "noisy" color display that detracts from the image quality and the diagnostic information. This occurs in approximately 20% of the adult patient population. One distracting artefact which is specific to some color flow instruments is widespread coloration of tissue areas of the image. These areas should only be displayed in gray scale since they contain no moving blood. However, if these tissue areas (valves, myocardium) are themselves moving, they may also generate a Doppler shift which the instrument then color codes accordingly. This artefact has been reduced in some instruments by the use of a subtraction processing algorithm which only displays color data in none tissue areas and a filtering system based upon a "moving target indicator principle". This latter technology is based upon World War II radar techniques!

Since color flow mapping is essentially a pulsed Doppler system, it suffers the same limitations in terms of the maximum flow velocity that can be detected without aliasing. In fact, the aliasing velocity is usually considerably lower with color flow mapping than conventional pulsed Doppler. When aliasing occurs, the colors are ambiguously displayed so that multiple colors appear in the flow jet. This is often described as a mosaic appearance. In theory, the fact that aliasing occurs at relatively low blood velocities (in relation to the transducer) is a disadvantage. In practice, this phenomenon is quite useful. Aliasing is very easy to identify in an image by the presence of the multiple colors. Therefore one's eye is drawn to areas of higher and possibly turbulent blood flow so that abnormalities are usually easy to detect. Examples of aliasing are seen in Plates 11.1 and 11.2.

It is important to remember that the blood velocity and direction displayed by the instrument is velocity and direction in relation to the transducer. For example, an aortic regurgitant jet may be moving slightly away from the transducer when viewed in the parasternal long axis view and will therefore be colored blue with some aliasing through to red, depending on the relative velocity, as shown in Plate 11.2. If the same jet is viewed from an apical position, it will now be moving toward the transducer with a higher relative velocity. In this case the jet will be colored red; however, there is likely to be multiple aliasing through to blue so that the flow jet will have a mosaic appearance. If a variance map is selected, then green will also be seen within the regurgitant jet (in either view), indicating that it is turbulent. This dependence on the relationship between the direction of the flow jet and the transducer may be confusing at first. The problem is being addressed by several manufacturers, so that future systems will utilize the jet direction and display flow colors that are dependent upon the true and not the relative blood velocity.

Applications

As with all Doppler techniques, color flow mapping requires a good understanding of, and ability to perform, conventional ultrasound imaging. However, no real additional skill is required to obtain satisfactory color flow images and the standard 2D imaging planes are usually utilized. The technique is at present qualitative rather than quantitative and it is unnecessary to "line up" with the flow as with conventional Doppler.

The first commercial color flow instruments suffered from a lack of sensitivity when compared with conventional Doppler. This was certainly a disadvantage, since it was possible to miss small, low volume flow jets. However, with improvements in technology, current instruments now have a sensitivity comparable to conventional pulsed Doppler. Continuous wave Doppler, using a dedicated Doppler rather than an imaging transducer, has the best sensitivity of all. In practice though, because color flow mapping scans most of the field of view, small elusive jets are comparatively easy to detect. The human eye is very good at pattern recognition and it is not difficult to recognize abnormal flow. These small jets may be missed by continuous or pulsed wave Doppler without detailed and somewhat tedious searching. However, the majority of these trivial flow jets are probably of little clinical significance.

The flow jets arising from ventricular septal defects can be very difficult to detect with conventional Doppler since they may be both small and eccentric. Furthermore, in patients with multiple defects, one or more of these may be missed entirely. Since small ventricular septal defect jets are almost always high velocity and turbulent, they are usually easy to detect within the color flow scan plane by the presence of aliasing (mosaic pattern) and variance (green color). Conventional continuous wave examination to record the jet velocity may then be performed, guided by the color flow map. An example of flow through a small muscular ventricular septal defect is seen in Plate 11.3.

Similar situations exist in patients with prosthetic valves, where regurgitant jets (valvular or paravalvar) are frequently very eccentric and difficult to document with conventional Doppler. However, confusing color flow artefacts may arise from the valve clicks and, in addition, shadowing by the prosthetic valve may make it difficult to detect regurgitant jets in some views. Nevertheless, some encouraging reports have suggested that prosthetic valve assessment is both easier and quicker when color flow mapping is used instead of conventional pulsed Doppler.

Regurgitant lesions in native valves are easy to detect with color flow mapping and several studies have reported a high sensitivity and specificity. Quantification of severity, with angiography as the gold standard, has been less successful. The correlation appears similar to that obtained with conventional Doppler. Superficially, angiography and color flow mapping may appear to provide similar types of flow images. However the source data is of course very different. Using angiography, the severity of regurgitation is usually graded qualitatively by assessing the extent of opacification and clearance time of the contrast medium from the receiving chamber, while color flow mapping demonstrates the spatial extent of the regurgitant jet velocities. Since these two techniques are actually measuring different parameters, frequently under different conditions, it is not surprising that the correlation is somewhat disappointing. Several color flow quantification techniques have been proposed, including planimetry of the area of the regurgitant jet, and measurement of its length and also the width near the origin. Unfortunately, all these parameters are influenced by a number of factors, including the sensitivity of the instrument, the gain settings, the view used, the regurgitant jet driving pressure and the precise part of the cardiac cycle in which the measurements are made. Despite these problems, the technique is more sensitive than auscultation, much easier to perform than angiography, and can usually separate regurgitant lesions into the clinically relevant categories of mild, moderate or severe.

One of the major limitations of conventional Doppler is that it does not facilitate appreciation of the spatial orientation of blood flow jets in the same way that color flow mapping does. For example, in cases of combined mitral stenosis and aortic regurgitation it can be difficult to separate the two diastolic flow jets in the left ventricle using conventional Doppler. Also, in patients with prosthetic valves and following mitral valvuloplasty the flow patterns may be very complicated and will often consist of multiple jets that cannot be appreciated or evaluated using pulsed Doppler. Other examples exist in patients with congenital cardiac lesions where there may be complex, multiple intracardiac shunts. In Plate 11.4 an example of severe mitral and tricuspid regurgitation is seen. The spatial extent of these regurgitant jets would have been very difficult to evaluate using conventional pulsed Doppler.

Color flow mapping may also assist and simplify quantitative flow velocity measurements made with conventional Doppler. For example, it is very easy to identify on the color flow map where the point of highest flow velocity is and then position the pulsed Doppler sample volume accordingly. This makes it unnecessary to search for the highest velocity point by repeatedly moving the pulsed Doppler sample volume.

The spatial direction of a flow jet is almost impossible to predict accurately using imaging and conventional Doppler. However, if reliable quantitative measurements are to be made, it is clearly important that the jet direction is known so that the orientation of the Doppler beam may be adjusted accordingly. There are many instances where color flow mapping may help to reduce the angle of incidence between the jet and the Doppler beam and therefore improve the accuracy of velocity and derived hemodynamic data. Examples include aortic stenosis, mitral stenosis, prosthetic mitral valves, ventricular septal defects and tricuspid regurgitation. In the latter case, it has been the experience of myself and others that improved prediction of pulmonary artery systolic pressure is possible if the continuous wave Doppler beam is aligned along the jet direction with color flow guidance. Some instruments which have the facility to perform continuous wave Doppler and color flow mapping utilizing the same transducer allow for angle correction to be made. However, it must be remembered that flow jets are three-dimensional and any angle correction can only possibly occur in one plane. Therefore it is better practice to minimize any angle of incidence by adjusting the position of the transducer and checking the jet direction in two orthogonal imaging planes.

Major patient management decisions are often made by cardiologists or surgeons who are unfamiliar with conventional Doppler spectral recordings and they may find color flow images easier to comprehend. In this way, the need for invasive investigation to document flow abnormalities before surgery may, in our experience, be reduced. For example, Plate 11.5 demonstrates a secundum atrial septal defect in which significant left-to-right shunting is clearly seen and further investigations prior to surgical closure were deemed unnecessary.

Transesophageal echocardiography is a relatively new echo modality which is currently attracting much attention. When this type of investigation is performed on conscious patients, a short examination time is of prime importance. For this reason, color flow mapping is now considered an essential adjunct to transesophageal echo.

Color flow mapping is new and appears to have great potential. It makes Doppler examinations quicker and easier to perform, and the diagnosis more obvious. It is likely that the technique will ultimately replace standard pulsed Doppler except in a few specific situations. However, the precise hemodynamic information available from the continuous wave technique will certainly still be needed.

The information provided by Doppler complements standard echo data to such an extent that together the two techniques have become the most important weapons in the cardiologist's diagnostic armamentarium. The need for invasive investigation of most cardiac lesions is now almost completely limited to delineation of the coronary anatomy, so that, despite the expense of providing trained, experienced staff and high quality echo/Doppler equipment, the techniques are extremely cost-effective.

Index